ISADORE ROSENFELD, M.D.

LIVE NOW AGE LATER

Proven Ways to Slow Down the Clock

WARNER BOOKS

A Time Warner Company

WARNER BOOKS EDITION

Copyright © 1999 by Isadore Rosenfeld, M.D.

Cover design by Flag

Warner Books, Inc.
1271 Avenue of the Americas
New York, NY 10020

Visit our Web site at
www.twbookmark.com

 A Time Warner Company

Printed in the United States of America

Originally published in hardcover by Warner Books.
First Paperback Printing: May 2000

10 9 8 7 6 5 4 3 2 1

ACCLAIM FOR *LIVE NOW, AGE LATER*

"Wise, practical, and essential reading. Only Dr. Rosenfeld can bring us the cutting-edge news on how to slow down aging and avoid many of its woes altogether."
—**Gail Sheehy, author of *Understanding Men's Passages***

"Genial, straight-talking . . . smart insights . . . refreshing honesty."   —*New York Daily News*

"Most welcome—the premise should get to every person concerned about getting older. . . . Many people are in need of Dr. Rosenfeld's counsel."
—**Hugh Downs, former correspondent, ABC's 20/20**

"Growing old doesn't have to be painful. . . . A genial, straight-talking, alphabetical rundown on the ills and side effects of age."   —*Fort Lauderdale Sun-Sentinel*

"A comprehensive, medically factual work that is highly readable, sprinkled with humor, and of great value to our aging population."
—**Michael E. DeBakey, M.D., Distinguished Service Professor and Olga Keith Weiss Professor of Surgery, Baylor College of Medicine**

"Excellent, comprehensive, very readable. . . . I recommend this book with enthusiasm."
—**Louis W. Sullivan, M.D., president, Morehouse School of Medicine, and former U.S. Secretary of Health and Human Services**

To my Camilla—
"Grow old along with me!"

And to our Anna Camilla
(born October 23, 1998)—
"The best is yet to be . . ."

ACKNOWLEDGMENTS

I am indebted to my colleagues who have reviewed the chapters specific to their expertise for accuracy. If you're unhappy about any of the information in the book, blame me, *not* them.

Denise Barbut, M.D.
Professor of Neurology
Director of Stroke Program, New York Presbyterian
Hospital/Weill School of Medicine, Cornell University

Murk-Hein Heinemann, M.D.
Chairman, Department of Ophthalmology, Memorial
Sloan-Kettering Cancer Center
Professor of Ophthalmology, New York Presbyterian
Hospital/Weill School of Medicine, Cornell University

Mark Pochapin, M.D.
Clinical Assistant Professor of Medicine and Associate
Chairman of Educational Affairs, New York
Presbyterian Hospital/Weill School of Medicine, Cornell
University

Marilyn Karmason, M.D.
Clinical Associate Professor, New York Presbyterian
Hospital/Weill School of Medicine, Cornell University

Shain Schley, M.D.
Chairman of Department of Otolaryngology, Cornell
University Medical College
Otorhinolaryngologist in Chief, New York Presbyterian
Hospital/Weill School of Medicine, Cornell University

Jean-Francois Eid, M.D.
Associate Professor of Urological Surgery, New York
Presbyterian Hospital/Weill School of Medicine, Cornell
University

Lawrence Kagen, M.D.
Professor of Medicine, New York Presbyterian
Hospital/Weill School of Medicine, Cornell University

Jason Lee, D.D.S.
Clinical Assistant Professor of Surgery (Dental and
Oral) and Attending Dentist, New York Presbyterian
Hospital/Weill School of Medicine, Cornell University

Robert Greenberg, M.D.
Assistant Clinical Professor, NYU Medical School

Maximilian Fink, M.D.
Professor of Psychiatry, Albert Einstein College of
Medicine
Professor Emeritus, SUNY Stony Brook

Holly S. Andersen, M.D.
Assistant Professor of Medicine, New York Presbyterian
Hospital/Weill School of Medicine, Cornell University

John Reckler, M.D.
Clinical Associate Professor of Urology, New York
Presbyterian Hospital/Weill School of Medicine, Cornell
University

CONTENTS

INTRODUCTION

> All the world's a stage,
> And all the men and women merely players;
> They have their exits and their entrances;
> And one man in his time plays many parts,
> His acts being seven ages. . . .
> Last scene of all,
> That ends this strange eventful history,
> Is second childishness and mere oblivion,
> Sans teeth, sans eyes, sans taste, sans everything.
> —WILLIAM SHAKESPEARE, *As You Like It*

Shakespeare was an astute observer. I have no doubt that most elderly people in his day were, in fact, "sans everything," but times have changed. Just look around you. Although Shakespeare's description does apply to some older folks, the majority are not edentulous, blind, or demented. And they function very well indeed.

My purpose in writing this book was not to tell you how great it is to grow old. I have too much respect for you to have titled it "Forever Young," or "The Golden Years," or "The Joys of Aging." No one remains young forever; the later years are rarely golden, and the most important joy of aging, as far as I am concerned, is grandchildren, if you're lucky enough to have them. Of course, maturity does bring wisdom and freedom from some of the less rational impulses that drove us when we were young. Many of us appreciate the filter of experience that shows us more clearly what really is important and worthy of our time and ambition—and what isn't. With many of our options diminished, we derive more pleasure from what we can do and have, rather than pine wistfully for what can never be. Still, I don't know anyone who wouldn't like to stop the clock. Unfortunately, that can't be done. If you live long enough, you will probably become infirm and develop at least some of the "trappings" of old age. However, you can make that happen later rather than sooner; you can delay the onset of disability and chronic disease so as to enjoy life and remain vigorous and independent for most of your later years. The goal of this book is to help you do just that. As you will see, in addition to a healthy lifestyle—whose components you already know, such as regular exercise; a diet low in fat and high in fish, fruits, and vegetables; moderation in alcohol intake; and abstinence from tobacco—there are specific measures for each of the "complications" of aging.

What particular aspect of getting old do you dread

most? Is it Alzheimer's? Physical weakness? Impotence? Deafness? Blindness? Cancer? Stroke? Heart trouble? Every one of these disorders, and many others, can be prevented, treated, or their progress slowed. But you can't sit back, leave it all to your doctor, and hope for the best. *You* are the key player on the team. In the following chapters you will read exactly what you must do to cope successfully with the biology of aging, when to start, and how to do it. I can't promise that you won't develop cancer, but you will learn how to reduce your chances of developing it; I can't guarantee that you won't have a stroke, but you'll know how to lessen that prospect by at least 50 percent; I can't stop you from tripping and falling, but there are ways to strengthen your bones so that you don't fracture them should you do so; and there are steps everyone should take that can decrease the chances of developing Alzheimer's. You will also learn how to reduce the risk of developing cataracts, overcome impotence, prevent and correct the wrinkling of your skin, maintain and improve muscle strength and balance, keep your own teeth longer than Shakespeare did—and much more.

Of course, there are those lucky few with the right genes who pay little or no attention to a healthy lifestyle and still enjoy a long life, right up to the very end. Winston Churchill is a prime example of such a health ne'er-do-well. He was overweight and stressed; he smoked like a chimney and drank like a fish; yet he lived life to the fullest into his nineties. Most of us, however, have to work at attaining healthy longevity.

The anti-aging "formula" for each of the disorders and symptoms discussed in this book is relevant to you no matter how old or how young you are because the aging process begins the moment you're born. The earlier you start preparing for it, the better. How you were fed as an infant, as well as the kind of lifestyle you adopt in your teens, twenties, and thirties, will determine the way you feel years down the line.

Each chapter deals with a specific complication of aging. But remember, I am not there to fasten your seat belt, to see that you wait for the green light before crossing, to stop you from jaywalking, and prevent you from driving after you drink. These are all things for which you are personally responsible. But barring such behavior, I believe that the practical advice in these pages will prolong your life, and allow you to enjoy it, too.

The author of any how-to book should be credible to his or her readers. Would you heed warnings about smoking from a doctor with a cigarette dangling from his lips? Would you take seriously any advice on how to stay thin from someone who weighs 300 pounds? Would you have confidence in recommendations on how to prevent going bald from someone who looks like Yul Brynner? By the same token, would you follow my advice on how to stay young if I myself appear to be prematurely old? I wanted to have my photograph on the cover of this book so that you could see that I don't look a day over 50. For some reason, I was advised not to do so! You'll have to take my word for it.

LIVE NOW
AGE
LATER

1

ALZHEIMER'S DISEASE

Remembering!

Any discussion of aging with someone older than fifty invariably makes them anxious about eventually losing their "marbles." Most of the other devastating ailments of mankind—cancer, heart trouble, stroke, even AIDS—don't usually produce the kind of terror associated with Alzheimer's disease. Cancer is certainly something to worry about, but it can often be detected early enough to be cured; its symptoms can be controlled, and patients may survive for months or even years. Everyone knows someone who has "conquered" a malignancy or coped with it for a long time. Stroke is also viewed with more equanimity these days; it can be prevented by effective treatment of high blood pressure; the likelihood of it causing permanent paralysis is not nearly as great as it used to be, thanks to sophisticated new medications and physical rehabilitation techniques. Proper diet, cholesterol-lowering drugs, and aspirin can prevent or delay heart disease. And if these measures don't work, there is a host of new procedures to treat most cardiac conditions: angioplasty, bypass surgery, valve replacement, laser beams directed into heart muscle, and gene therapy that forms new blood vessels. As a last resort, there's the option of a heart transplant. Even the outlook for AIDS has improved. New drugs prolong life and improve its quality among those afflicted, and HIV infections sometimes even disappear spontaneously.

I am not suggesting that these illnesses always end happily, but they rarely have the emotional impact of chronic dementia. When your mind is intact, you retain some control over your life; you can try to cope with adversity; you can make decisions about your care; you can plan; you can still hope. You have your soul. None of this is true for Alzheimer's disease. Most victims eventually end up in a vegetative state, totally estranged from their environment and unable to communicate with or even recognize their closest loved ones. Tragically, many of them are physically strong enough to hang on to "life" for twenty years or more, during which time the strain on family and friends is unrelenting and unbearable.

Close blood relatives of Alzheimer's patients naturally worry about their own long-term outlook, and for good reason. They read into every minor memory lapse the portents of the disease; they panic when they can't remember a name or where they've put their car keys—even though such lapses are experienced now and then by everyone at every age.

Alzheimer's *is* a terrible disease, for which there is no

cure. Although its rate of progress varies, the road is inexorably downhill. However, there *are* things you can do, and medications you *can* take, to delay or possibly even prevent its onset. The sooner you start them, the better.

The Alzheimer's Brain

Until the early 1900s, people believed that if they lived long enough they would inevitably develop "senile dementia" and that losing their mind was a normal accompaniment of aging. But in 1906 a German neuropathologist named Alois Alzheimer looked under the microscope at the brains of relatively young "demented" people who had died in their fifties and sixties. He noted that there were areas in which the nerve fibers had lost their normal orderly appearance and become all tangled up. He termed this disarray "neurofibrillary tangles" and believed that they were only present in young persons who were prematurely deranged. So for many years, doctors limited the diagnosis of "Alzheimer's disease" to young people who were demented. We now know that the brains of elderly persons with "senile dementia" also have these twisted fibers. (They are also occasionally present in other neurological disorders such as Lou Gehrig's disease—amyotrophic lateral sclerosis—and Down's syndrome.) In other words, Alzheimer's is a disease that can occur at any age and is not an inevitable accompaniment of aging.

What Causes Alzheimer's Disease?

The cause of Alzheimer's disease—why these neurofibrillary tangles develop in some people and not in others—remains a mystery. Modern methods of analyzing brain tissue have revealed that the neurofibrillary tangles are deposits or plaques of abnormal proteins, the most common of which is beta amyloid. An Alzheimer's brain is also deficient in several neurotransmitters (chemicals that allow nerves in different parts of the brain to send messages to each other), the best known of which is acetylcholine. Although replenishing these neurotransmitters has no real impact on dementia, doing so sometimes alleviates symptoms.

There are several interesting theories about the cause of Alzheimer's. One suggests that the culprit is an as yet unidentified virus. Or perhaps the brain may be deficient in nerve growth factor (NGF), a substance that stimulates the formation of new nerve connections (synapses). When the brain is lacking in NGF and can't make enough synapses, memory and intellectual function become impaired. When NGF is administered to rats, new connections form in those areas of the brain that are concerned with memory. Although these and other observations hold out the promise that Alzheimer's will one day be cured, don't hold your breath—at least for the moment.

Who's Vulnerable?

How do you know if you're especially susceptible to Alzheimer's? There are no absolute risk factors, but there are some statistical correlations.

• **Age:** Full-blown Alzheimer's affects about 4 million Americans, virtually all of whom are older than sixty; the majority are beyond eighty-five. At least half the current residents of nursing homes in this country have Alzheimer's disease; most of the others are there because they have brain damage from recurrent small strokes, Parkinson's disease, and other less common neurological disorders.

• **Family History:** The risk of getting Alzheimer's in your lifetime is slightly more if any of your close relatives, such as a parent, sibling, or child is, or was, affected. However, the more such relatives you have, the greater your risk. (In-laws don't count.)

• **Genetics:** A specific gene called ApoE, usually situated on chromosome #19, is a marker of susceptibility to Alzheimer's in about 15 percent of the population. However, if you happen to carry it, don't panic. Most persons who do never develop Alzheimer's, and vice versa. More recently, another gene, this one located on the #12 chromosome, has been found in up to 15 percent of late-onset Alzheimer's (appearing at or beyond age 80). Again, its presence merely indicates that, in combination with certain environmental factors, you may be predisposed to Alzheimer's but are by no means certain to develop it. Although genetic testing is important in the research of

Alzheimer's disease, it is not yet precise enough to warrant its routine use. It is not clear why Hispanics and Blacks without these specific genes are at two and four times the risk, respectively, of developing Alzheimer's disease. Some other as yet unidentified gene or genes, or perhaps environmental factors such as diet, occupation, and exposure to toxic substances, may be responsible.

Other possible causes of Alzheimer's that have been suggested but remain unproved include underactivity of the thyroid gland (hypothyroidism) and chronic alcohol excess.

Symptoms of Alzheimer's

Full-blown Alzheimer's impairs virtually every function of the brain: memory, behavior, abstract thinking, personality, judgment, language, movement, and coordination. It's interesting that patients with Alzheimer's lose these abilities in the reverse sequence in which we develop them during childhood. For example, the very first thing babies can do is swallow; then they recognize and respond to the mother or other caregiver; next they begin to repeat words; then they walk; next in the sequence are bladder and bowel control; finally they begin to converse, to exercise their memory, and to demonstrate judgment. In Alzheimer's, the higher thought processes are the first to go. The earliest symptoms are impaired learning and an inability to retain new information, lack of reasoning power, trouble performing complex tasks, a distinctive subtle change in personality, confusion, and a lack of orientation. These are followed by loss of bladder and bowel control, and walking is progressively more difficult. As motor skills become impaired, the Alzheimer's patient cannot walk unassisted, is unable to swallow normally, and often dies from pneumonia due to aspiration of fluid or liquid into the lung.

Make Sure It's Alzheimer's

Dementia is not always due to Alzheimer's. At least 20 percent of older people suffer from other conditions that mimic it, the most important of which are:

• **Depression:** When you're depressed, you're not terribly concerned with remembering details, learning new facts, mastering new skills, or socializing—criteria by which mental capacity is often judged. Lack of involvement and enthusiasm are often interpreted as evidence of Alzheimer's. In one of my other books, I recounted the story of a man whose children were convinced that he had Alzheimer's because he'd become withdrawn for no apparent reason. He was a widower who lived alone, and the family didn't think he was really able to care for himself. They decided he'd be better off in a "retirement" home. He agreed to move—or, rather, he didn't resist the decision because he couldn't care less where he lived or what he did. A few weeks after moving into the senior citizens' residence that had been chosen for him, he met a woman whose company he enjoyed. They fell in love and—presto—his "personality change" cleared up and his "Alzheimer's" disappeared. The couple married, moved out of the home, rented an apartment in the city, started visiting museums, went to the theater and movies, and developed a close circle of friends. So always think of depression before deciding someone has Alzheimer's.

• **Subdural hematoma** refers to a pocket of blood that has accumulated on the inside of the skull, usually as a result of a blow or other injury to the head. This damages blood vessels on the inner surface of the skull and makes them bleed. The blood that accumulates exerts pressure on the underlying brain, causing headache, personality changes, and a variety of other neurological symptoms. Because blood vessels are more fragile in older people, they tear more easily so that even a minor knock on the head can cause a subdural hematoma. This condition can be cured by either removing the blood clot with a needle or by shrinking it with steroid drugs.

Subdural hematomas are often unrecognized when the injury that caused them is trivial and not immediately followed by symptoms. Always suspect this possibility in any older person with an unexplained change in behavior or personality or a persistent headache. And when you do, get a CT scan of the brain to confirm the diagnosis. I remember one man who knocked his head on a shelf in his bathroom while looking for some aftershave lotion. The injury had left no bump, scar, or other mark, so he didn't tell anyone about it. A few weeks later his wife noticed that he was drowsy and confused. Probably Alzheimer's, she thought. After all, he was eighty! Yet he had always been so sharp. Why now? And why so suddenly? A CT scan revealed a large subdural hematoma from just this little bang on the head. It was removed with a needle, and the "Alzheimer's" was cured!

• **Multiple small strokes:** A *stroke* occurs when an area of the brain is suddenly deprived of its blood supply. This can happen in several ways: blockage of one or more of the arteries situated either within the brain or leading to it from the neck (thrombosis); when an artery in the brain bursts after being weakened by long-standing, untreated high blood pressure, or by a congenital abnormality of its wall (an aneurysm); or when the flow of blood in a brain artery is cut off by a clot that has made its way into the cerebral circulation from somewhere in the heart or neck vessels (embolism).

The symptoms of stroke (paralysis, impaired speech, blindness, loss of balance, incontinence), and their severity, depend on what caused it—a hemorrhage, a traveling blood clot, or a blockage. Was the involved vessel large or small? How much of the brain and what part of it was damaged or destroyed? Involvement of just a single small blood vessel usually results in only limited injury, and the symptoms are apt to be minor and transient. However, when such little strokes keep recurring, their cumulative effect can cause enough brain damage to produce memory loss and personality change. This train of events is referred to as multi-infarct dementia (*infarct* means death of tissue). We can often stop the progress of such dementia by preventing these strokes by dietary means, blood pressure control (so that blood vessels are not prematurely clogged by arteriosclerotic plaques), or blood thinning (either with aspirin or other anticoagulants). By contrast, the dementia of Alzheimer's disease usually progresses relentlessly.

• **Brain tumors,** which either originate in the brain itself or have spread to it from a distant site (a metastasis), are a much less frequent cause of dementia than are strokes or subdural hematomas. However, always think of a tumor in someone with otherwise unexplained neurological symptoms or behavioral changes. I remember a successful businessman in his middle fifties who was sent to a mental hospital with a diagnosis of Alzheimer's disease because he was becoming more and more irrational. Only at autopsy was the malignant brain tumor—the real cause of his symptoms—discovered.

• **Hypothyroidism:** The thyroid gland is the body's energy thermostat. When less thyroid hormone is produced (hypothyroidism), overall metabolism slows down: Your energy level decreases, your speech is less spontaneous, and your mental functions are not as sharp as they used to be.

Hypothyroidism can occur at any age, and it is not uncommon among the elderly. Unfortunately, even though it is easily diagnosed by means of a simple blood test, doctors and patients don't think of this possibility often enough. You have no idea how many patients I've seen over the years with typical complaints of hypothyroidism—inability to lose weight, constantly feeling cold, constipated, no energy, depressed, even confused—who went untreated for years because their mental sluggishness was mistaken for Alzheimer's. Always suspect thyroid underfunction in any older person who has slowed down both physically and mentally for no apparent reason. It's amazing how thyroid supplements will cure most of their symptoms, including their "dementia."

• **Alcohol and substance abuse:** Longtime alcohol use and abuse can damage the brain and cause behavioral changes that resemble Alzheimer's disease. It doesn't have to be excessive drinking, either. The amount of alcohol that can alter personality varies from person to person. You can recognize brain damage due to booze by other evidence of alcohol toxicity, such as a florid face and, in men, manifestations of feminization such as enlarged breasts, diminished facial hair, and loss of libido. However, when the same individual has both chronic alcoholism and Alzheimer's, it's not easy to tell which condition is causing what symptoms. None of the treatments that occasionally improve the symptoms of Alzheimer's (see below) have any impact on alcohol-induced dementia.

• **Polypharmacy** means taking a lot of drugs. Americans over seventy years of age consume an average of six or seven different pills every day, both over-the-counter and prescription (not to mention herbal remedies.) That's because doctors too often recommend a quick fix for whatever ails their older patients. Trouble sleeping? Take this sedative. Tired? Try this "pick-me-up." Have a cold? Use this antibiotic. Suffering from arthritic pains? These painkillers will help. No appetite? Here are some great multivitamins. Anxious? This tranquilizer will help relax you.

Sedatives, sleeping pills, tranquilizers, and painkillers are the agents most likely to affect behavior. However, any drug or combination of drugs taken for any purpose can produce personality changes and memory loss. For example, you wouldn't think that a drug to treat urinary incontinence could impair memory. Yet in one study, 10 milligrams daily of oxybutynin chloride (Ditropan), widely prescribed for this disorder, affected language and mental performance. Since incontinence most commonly occurs in older persons, you can imagine a scenario in which someone using Ditropan might be thought to have early Alzheimer's. Identifying and withdrawing the offending agent, whatever it is, can result in a miraculous cure of "Alzheimer's"!

• **Malnutrition** is perhaps the most common cause, aside from Alzheimer's, of behavioral changes in the elderly. Every organ in the body, including the brain, can malfunction when you don't eat nutritious foods for whatever reason: because you've lost your teeth and can't chew; you're alone, depressed, or just can't be bothered to cook for yourself; you can't afford to buy the food you need; or some medication you're taking is killing your appetite. Normal mental function has been restored in countless older people with "Alzheimer's disease" after they were given nutritious meals and vitamin supplements. (That's why I prescribe a multivitamin supplement to every senior citizen who lives alone.)

• **Other underlying diseases,** acute or chronic, can produce behavioral changes at any age, especially in the elderly. Is it any wonder that a mind doesn't function normally in someone with emphysema in whom the effort of just breathing wears them out? Or if the heart isn't pumping enough blood and oxygen to the brain? Or if the kidneys have stopped working and toxins are accumulating in the body? Behavior mimicking Alzheimer's can also develop when the brain is physically injured in an accident, directly infected by some virus or fungus, or exposed to poisons such as carbon monoxide or methyl alcohol.

Diagnosing Alzheimer's

There is no reliable marker that identifies Alzheimer's with certainty during life. Even the most sophisticated scans cannot reveal the neurofibrillary tangles or the amyloid plaques in someone who's still alive. An abnormal protein called Alzheimer's Disease Associated Protein (ADAP) has recently been found only in the brains of persons who have died with Alzheimer's. Hopefully, scientists will one day develop a test that can identify this protein in the spinal fluid or blood during life and so diagnose Alzheimer's clinically. At the present time, however, doctors make the diagnosis only after all other possible causes of dementia have been eliminated.

Because of these limitations, Alzheimer's is the most overdiagnosed and misdiagnosed mental ailment in older people. Whenever this disorder is suspected, a thorough examination must be done to eliminate all other possibilities. This should include, in addition to

the physical itself, a careful and detailed history to identify any family predisposition. It's important also to in-
vestigate the possibility of poor nutrition, a head injury,
the use or abuse of medication, or the presence of other
medical problems.

An evaluation of mental status and neuropsychological
testing are also in order. Most family doctors are not
trained to do so, and even if they are they would usually
recommend a specialist, such as a neurologist, psychologist, or psychiatrist. No screening for Alzheimer's is
complete without an electroencephalogram (EEG) to an-
alyze the brain waves, and a CT scan of the brain to visualize its physical structure. Magnetic resonance
imaging (MRI) and positron emission tomography
(PET), which provide data concerning the metabolic activity of the brain and cerebral function, are expensive
and rarely necessary. Ask a good neurologist to decide
what special procedures, if any, are necessary.

How to Reduce Your Chances of Getting Alzheimer's

Despite the absence of a cure for Alzheimer's, there are
some proven ways to help your brain stay young and
lessen your chances of developing this disease.

• **Ongoing mental and physical exercise** keep the
brain healthy. Either "use it or lose it." Regular physical
activity increases blood flow to the brain and provides the
nutrients necessary to render its tissues resistant to

Alzheimer's. Exercise also increases the number of connections (synapses) among the millions of brain cells (neurons) needed for normal mental function. In a recent experiment on laboratory rats, performance was compared in two groups: controls, given no opportunity to play or exercise; and a "treated" group, provided with toys and made to exercise vigorously. After a few weeks, the brains of the treated animals were found to have 25 percent more connections (synapses) than the couch potatoes. Get into the habit of walking for thirty to sixty minutes a day as briskly as possible. Stair climbing is particularly effective, so take the steps when going up or down one or two flights and leave the elevators and escalators to the kids.

• **Education:** Several population studies have shown that the more schooling you have, the greater are your chances against Alzheimer's. That may be because the educated are more likely to eat more nutritiously and receive better medical care throughout their lives. However, like physical exercise, ongoing intellectual challenges stimulate the formation of nerve connections. Even if you're destined to develop Alzheimer's, the more neurons you develop when you're young, the more you can afford to lose before symptoms set in. This theory is supported by the observation that symptoms of Alzheimer's disease in persons whose head circumference is greater than twenty-four inches—and who therefore have a greater brain mass—progress more slowly than they do in "pinheads." So calling someone a "fathead" may actually be a compliment!

Many retired seniors sign up for classes in accounting, law, art, music, economics, or whatever else interests them to stay mentally active, and not necessarily to start a second career. The longer you continue your education at any age, or keep your mind busy in some other way, the more likely your neurons are to connect with each other later on.

• **Reaction to stress:** Stress is blamed for almost everything that goes wrong in life: "I can't sleep, I'm under too much stress." "My job is too stressful for me to do it right." "My bowels aren't moving right. You know how much stress I'm under." "My marriage is on the rocks. It's the stress, you know." Although stress is a convenient scapegoat, it probably does play a role in the development of Alzheimer's. The body reacts to stress by producing extra amounts of cortisol, a hormone that shrinks the hippocampus, the area in the brain that controls memory and interferes with its normal function. The calmer and more self-confident you are in a crisis, whether it is short-lived or prolonged, the less cortisol is produced.

• **Diet:** Eat as little animal fat as possible to reduce your vulnerability to Alzheimer's. The incidence of Alzheimer's in different countries correlates with the consumption of total fat. For example, in the United States, 5 percent of all persons over the age of sixty-five have the disease, while in China and Nigeria, where the fat intake is much lower, the incidence is only 1 percent. Japanese who move to America and double the amount of fat in their diet have twice the incidence of Alzheimer's than do those who do not emigrate and presumably maintain their old eating habits.

Here is another dietary tip: The more fish you eat, the less likely you are to get Alzheimer's. That's because the neurofibrillary tangles and amyloid plaques may, at least in part, be due to inflammation within the brain. The protective effect of fish is probably due to the anti-inflammatory properties of Omega-3 fatty acids, present in highest concentrations in deep-sea, cold-water fish such as mackerel, tuna, halibut, and sardines. Eat at least three to six ounces of these fish every week. If you don't like seafood, or can't afford it, you can obtain Omega-3 fatty acids in capsule form. Make sure to get a "reputable" brand, since some of the commercial preparations can turn rancid. I prefer the fish.

Holistic practitioners believe that several foods are "brain builders." For example, they claim that artichokes increase mental acuity; brewers' yeast makes for better brain function; sardines, rich in coenzyme Q10, raise the concentration of cerebral oxygen; lettuce, raw or juiced, which is rich in iron and magnesium, builds brain cells; and parsnip—raw, juiced, or in salad—improves cognition. I know of no scientific documentation for any of these assertions, but why not try them? My mother, who was not a holistic practitioner, always recommended them, as I'm sure yours did too.

• If you're menopausal, ask your doctor about **estrogen replacement therapy (ERT)**. It's safe for most women, except for those with a blood-clotting problem or a history of a hormone-related cancer (breast, uterus, or ovaries). Recent studies of thousands of women seventy years of age and older have shown that estrogen replacement therapy improves short-term memory and increases the capacity to learn and retain new facts. Fewer women who have taken this hormone for at least one year end up with Alzheimer's, and those who have been on it for ten or more years have a 40 to 54 percent lower incidence of developing the disease than those who haven't. These are impressive figures, and they make a strong case for such replacement therapy. How estrogen protects against Alzheimer's is not clear, but it probably stimulates the neurons to form new connections. The National Institutes of Health is currently conducting a study of 8,000 healthy women sixty-five years of age or older who are on estrogen to further document this hormone's effect on the development of Alzheimer's. Don't wait for the results. Take estrogen now, especially if you are worried about Alzheimer's.

• **Nonsteroidal anti-inflammatory drugs (NSAIDs):** Millions of us use these drugs for relief of everything from headache to arthritis. Some of the more popular brands are Nuprin, Advil, Aleve, Motrin, Anaprox, Naprosyn, Oruvail, and Relafen. Several years ago, researchers noted a 50 percent lower incidence of Alzheimer's in persons with rheumatoid arthritis who had been using these drugs for any length of time. In a study of identical twins, those who took anti-inflammatory drugs had a lower incidence of the disease than their siblings who did not. Alzheimer's patients who take daily aspirin or other NSAIDs have better verbal and mental functioning scores too, and the rate of their overall deterioration is measurably slower.

A maintenance dose of NSAIDs may slow the progression of Alzheimer's, but it can cause subtle intestinal bleeding, as well as kidney and liver problems. Two other drugs that may work in a similar way are currently being studied. The first, colchicine, is used mainly in the prevention and treatment of acute gout; the other, chloroquine, is an antimalarial drug. It's too early to recommend either of these agents for the management of Alzheimer's.

• **Nicotine** is a prime example of how new research data can supersede and negate previously acquired information. We used to believe that smokers were less likely than nonsmokers to develop Alzheimer's. But the antitobacco community is now breathing easier (no pun intended) because more recent studies indicate that smoking actually doubles the risk of getting Alzheimer's.

• **Vitamin E:** Hardly a day goes by without some favorable report about vitamin E. I can't think of any downside to this vitamin, with the possible exception of its raising blood pressure and causing some "extra beats" in some people. Vitamin E increases fertility in rats (which is why it was originally dubbed the "fertility" vitamin); it's good for the heart; and many doctors prescribe it for the treatment of vascular disease, particularly for narrowing the arteries in the legs. Now comes word that vitamin E may also delay the onset of Alzheimer's, presumably by virtue of its antioxidant properties. Antioxidants, of which there are many (such as vitamin C and selenium), are said to neutralize the harmful effects of free radicals, the byproducts of bodily processes that involve oxygen. These radicals carry an extra electron that can damage the protein in the brain and other organs and accelerate the aging process. The body's own antioxidants normally neutralize these free radicals, but this defense can be enhanced by supplemental vitamin E. Although most doctors recommend 400 to 800 international units per day, researchers at the University of California in San Diego observed maximum effects from a daily dosage of 2,000 i.u. in persons with Alzheimer's.

• **Choline** is a building block for acetylcholine, the neurotransmitter in short supply in Alzheimer's patients. Choline and other drugs that raise acetylcholine levels in the brain (lecithin, physostigmine, deprenyl), used alone or in combination are hot items in pharmacies and health food stores. They are sold for the prevention and treatment of Alzheimer's disease. I am not impressed with the evidence documenting the claims made for any of them, and I have never seen any beneficial effects from their use in my own practice. Some proponents of choline contend that young people should be taking it before the brain is damaged. There's no downside to doing so as a preventive, assuming you have the money to spend on what may turn out to be a waste. Most of the twenty new "cognition-enhancing" drugs now being evaluated in human subjects potentiate or mimic the effects of acetylcholine.

• Neurofibrillary tangles found at autopsy have an unusually high **aluminum** content. Some doctors believe that this metal causes Alzheimer's, and they recommend avoiding it whenever possible. That means no aluminum-containing deodorants and no aluminum-rich antacids. Most experts, however, doubt that aluminum is the villain. They are of the opinion that it is deposited after the fact in areas that have previously been damaged by the Alzheimer's process. Although I am not personally convinced that aluminum plays a role in Alzheimer's, I try to keep away from it anyway because I'd rather be safe than sorry. It's easy enough to use pots and pans that don't give off aluminum and to avoid antacids that contain it. But, frankly, when my heartburn gets really bad, I capitulate and take whatever will give me relief—whether or not it contains aluminum.

Treating Alzheimer's

The symptoms of Alzheimer's disease can remain mild for a long time, so that many of those afflicted can continue to function at home with relatively little care from others. However, as the disease progresses, most patients eventually require total care—feeding, dressing, and constant monitoring.

Although there is no specific treatment for Alzheimer's, every patient should be given a good multivitamin because his or her diet can be so unpredictable. I also recommend at least 120 milligrams of *Ginkgo biloba* daily. Ginkgo is an herb that is said to increase blood flow to the brain, heart, and extremities. Reports from Europe and Asia have attested to its effectiveness in improving memory in older people. The American medical literature on the efficacy of ginkgo has been sparse—until now. In 1997 doctors at the New York Institute for Medical Research reported in the *Journal of the American Medical Association* that an extract of ginkgo stabilized, and in some cases improved, the cognitive function and the social behavior of demented persons for six months to a year. This was not the anecdotal type of study criticized by scientifically trained doctors but a double-blind, placebo-controlled, parallel-group multicenter trial.

Ginkgo has few if any side effects and is worth trying. But remember that it interacts with and enhances the effect of blood thinners such as aspirin or Coumadin, and that the dose of these two drugs may have to be reduced if you're also taking ginkgo.

Tacrine (Cognex) and *donepezil* (Aricept) are now specifically marketed for the treatment of Alzheimer's. They inhibit the enzyme (acetylcholinesterase) that breaks down acetylcholine in the brain. Both these agents can result in some temporary memory improvement. They're worth trying.

What to Remember about Alzheimer's

1. Alzheimer's is a distinct disease of unknown cause that ultimately leads to dementia. It is not an inevitable accompaniment of aging.

2. The diagnosis of Alzheimer's is one of exclusion. There is no test currently available to make the diagnosis during life. This can only be done with certainty by examining the brain after death.

3. A family history of Alzheimer's only slightly increases your risk of developing the disease.

4. Several genes associated with Alzheimer's have been identified. However, people who harbor them may never develop the disease, which may also strike those who don't have them.

5. Alzheimer's is frequently overdiagnosed and misdiagnosed in older people because there are many different diseases and disorders that can mimic its symptoms and cause dementia. Unlike Alzheimer's, some of these other conditions are preventable and curable. The diagnosis of Alzheimer's should never be made without a thorough and complete neurological examination.

6. Lifestyle changes, including a low-fat diet, education, and exercise, can lower the risk of Alzheimer's.

7. Several agents, including antioxidants, anti-inflammatory drugs, hormones, ginkgo, and vitamin E, may reduce the chances of developing Alzheimer's.

8. There is only a handful of drugs on the market for the treatment of the established form of the disease, none of which are very effective. Supportive care remains the basic treatment of Alzheimer's.

2

CANCER

Of Mice and Men

Cancer is responsible for the second largest number of deaths in this country (just behind heart disease, and somewhat ahead of stroke). It claims 550,000 lives a year, and 55 percent of these deaths are due to the four major cancers: lung, colon/rectum, breast, and prostate. (Although skin cancer is the most common malignancy, it's not one of the major killers.)

Cancer is a terrible disease. The very word strikes terror into the hearts of most people. I have patients and friends who will never even utter it, as if just doing so might in some way endanger them. No one is immune to cancer. Although the right genes and a healthy lifestyle leave you somewhat less vulnerable, they do not guarantee that you will not be stricken.

Despite all the media hype about "breakthroughs," many cancers remain incurable unless they're detected early. There's nothing more frustrating and stressful for the loved ones (and doctor) of a dying cancer patient than to witness such pain and suffering, to be helpless to alter the relentless course, and at the same time to feel constrained to hold out hope when none exists. On the bright side, dedicated researchers continue their intense efforts with zeal and optimism. As you've probably heard in the media, they're doing great things for cancerous mice, some of which they hope will also benefit humans. In addition to the ongoing animal research, the following list shows the number of medications and vaccines being tested in 1998 on people on this country alone:

- Skin cancer—60
- Breast cancer—59
- Lung cancer—42
- Prostate cancer—36
- Colorectal cancer—35
- Leukemia—35
- Lymphoma—33
- Ovarian cancer—24
- Cancers of the head and neck—18

Until the researchers come up with something more dramatic, the best chance to cure cancer is to find it early enough. That's easier to do if you have a basic understanding of the disease.

How Cancers Start

When a body organ or tissue needs to replace cells that are worn out or have died, its healthy cells divide and increase in number. They do so in an orderly way, and produce no more cells than are necessary. The cells of cancerous tissue, on the other hand, multiply for no reason, and they do so like crazy, without rhyme or reason. Their lack of restraint is probably triggered by some damage to their DNA, which results in a change (mutation) of one or more critical genes. For example, uncontrolled cell division occurs when P53, a tumor suppressor gene whose job is to regulate cell division, is inactivated or mutated. So cancer *is a disease of the genes,* a malfunction of the proteins (DNA) in our chromosomes.

This exuberant cellular multiplication results in a "growth" or tumor that is either benign or malignant. When a tumor is benign, it stays in one place; its cells do not spread to other parts of the body; it rarely threatens life; and it almost never recurs after it's removed. Cancers, by contrast, invade and press on adjacent organs and tissues; their cells later break away from the parent growth (the primary), enter the bloodstream or the lymphatic system, and travel throughout the body, settling all over the place. This spread is called metastasis.

Cancer and Aging

Although cancer strikes both young and old, it is primarily a disease of aging. In the United States, 50 percent of all malignancies and 67 percent of cancer deaths occur in persons over the age of sixty-five. (That's currently one American in eight; by the year 2030, it's expected to be one in five.) Yet, even though they are ten times more likely than younger persons to develop cancer, the elderly are not screened as often; they're referred less frequently to major cancer centers where they have a better chance of being cured; and they're usually treated less aggressively for their disease.

Older people are more vulnerable to cancer because of their longer exposure to carcinogens: pollution, radiation, tobacco, sun, alcohol, the wrong diet, chemical or physical irritation, hormonal imbalance, and possibly even stress. Random genetic mutations that lead to cancer also occur more frequently. The body's DNA repair system, which is constantly on the lookout for dangerous changes that may cause a cell to become cancerous—and aborts the cell when such mutations are detected—is less effective as we grow older.

The outcome of cancer in many older persons is adversely affected by a combination of social, psychological, educational, financial, cultural, and economic factors. The elderly are not always aware of all the hows, whys, and wheres of cancer diagnosis and therapy because much of the pertinent educational material is not geared toward them. As a result, they may assume that all cancers are uniformly fatal, and that there's nothing to be done about them. They may attribute their symptoms to some other cause, or to "old age," and they put off seeing a doctor until it's too late. They may have legitimate concerns about their ability to pay for the care they need, especially since many services, such as outpatient drugs, transportation, home care, and medical supplies, are not covered by Medicare. Some of my elderly patients have refused expensive procedures and not filled their prescriptions because they couldn't afford them. If they live in social isolation, without a strong support network of family, friends, and neighbors, they may not be able to get to the clinic or the doctor's office because they don't have a car or can't drive, or they have physical limitations. Finally, the chances of curing their cancer may be affected by a coexisting chronic illness, such as a respiratory problem, arthritis, diabetes, or heart trouble. Some or all of these factors are not always taken into account, given the medical establishment's preoccupation with profit, statistics, efficiency, and technology.

Preventing Cancer

A complex mix of factors related to environment, lifestyle, and heredity plays a role in the causation of cancer. For example, 80 percent of all cancers are related to the use of tobacco products, to what we eat and drink, and to our exposure to radiation, asbestos, and some of the other cancer-causing agents. There's not much you can do about your genes (at the moment), but several other key risk factors *are* under your control. If you identify them and make the necessary changes in your lifestyle early enough, you can substantially decrease your chances of developing a malignancy. Here are some of the risk factors you can do something about:

• **Tobacco** is the most preventable cause of mortality in this country. Regardless of whether you chew it, snuff it, smoke it, or inhale someone else's "exhaust" (passive smoking causes about 3,000 lung-cancer deaths every year), tobacco is a killer. In the United States, it is responsible for 85 to 90 percent of all lung cancers, and for one-third of all deaths related to other cancers (mouth, larynx, esophagus, stomach, pancreas, bladder, kidney, cervix, leukemia, and possibly colon). The magnitude of the risk depends on the number and kind of cigarettes you've smoked and for how long. A pack-a-day smoker is ten times more vulnerable than a nonsmoker. It's never too late to quit. After you do, your cancer risk declines gradually each year.

• **Chronic alcohol abuse** can cause cancer of the liver, as well as of the mouth, throat, esophagus, and larynx, especially in combination with tobacco. It may also raise the risk of breast cancer. If you're going to imbibe, limit yourself to the equivalent of two drinks a day—and stop smoking.

• **Diet:** People who shun fruits and vegetables have roughly twice the incidence of most types of cancer— lung, larynx, oral cavity, esophagus, stomach, colon and rectum, bladder, pancreas, cervix, and ovary—than those with the highest intake. Yet only 9 percent of Americans heed the recommendations of the National Cancer Institute and the National Research Council to eat two servings of fruit and three portions of vegetables a day. Seventh-Day Adventists, who don't drink or eat much meat but do consume a diet rich in fruits and vegetables, have the lowest incidence of cancer in the U.S. population. This protective effect is probably due to the antioxidants and folic acid present in fruits and vegetables, which neutralize damage to chromosomal DNA caused by oxygen-free radicals.

• **Some supplements** seem to protect against certain cancers. For instance, colon polyps and cancer do not recur as often in persons who regularly take multivitamins, calcium supplements, and vitamin E. And in a recent study conducted in England, a daily dose of 50 milligrams of vitamin E reduced the incidence of prostate cancer. However, you're usually better off with the natural sources from which these supplements are extracted, rather than getting them from a bottle. A diet rich in fruits and vegetables is protective against cancer, presumably because of the beta-carotene content. Yet in a now-famous Finnish study, beta-carotene supplements appeared to increase the risk of lung cancer (as well as coronary artery disease and total mortality). Researchers enlisted thousands of heavy smokers especially vulnerable to cancer. The subjects were divided into two groups—one was given placebos, and the other, beta-carotene. After a few years, the latter, surprisingly, were found to have a 17 percent higher incidence of lung cancer! So take your mother's advice: Eat all the fruits and vegetables you can—and forget the pills.

• **A high-fat diet** is associated with cancer of the breast, uterus, and prostate. The guilty foods are eggs, fatty meats, high-fat salad dressings and cooking oils, and dairy products such as whole milk, butter, and most cheeses.

Blueberries have a higher antioxidant capacity than any other fruit or vegetable. They are said to protect against cancer by virtue of their anthocyanins and other natural phytochemicals. (Anthocyanins give wild blueberries their intense blue color.)

• **A high consumption of soy-based food,** such as tofu, may also protect against cancer because of the genistein content. Genistein suppresses the production of proteins that cancer cells need in order to keep growing. In China and Japan, where people eat lots of soy, there is much less cancer of the breast, colon, and prostate than in this country. Since men with prostate cancer generally have lower blood levels of selenium than their normal counterparts, selenium supplements may protect against this malignancy.

• **Significant overweight** is linked to cancer of the prostate, pancreas, uterus, colon, ovary, and, in older women, the breast.

• **A low-calorie, low-protein diet** markedly decreases tumor incidence and increases life span in rats. Scientists are currently trying to decide whether these observations apply to humans, too.

In summary, I believe the ideal anticancer diet is one that's varied, well balanced, and includes at least five servings of fruits and vegetables each day; lots of grain, breads, and cereals (to provide the necessary fiber); and is as low in fat as possible.

• **Ultraviolet radiation** from sun, sunlamps, and tanning booths damages the skin and can cause skin cancer. Stay out of the bright sun between 11:00 a.m. and 3:00

p.m. (If you don't have a watch and are not sure of the time, avoid the sun when your shadow is shorter than you are.) If you must be in the sun during those hours, wear protective clothing (a hat, long sleeves) and apply sunblock with a protection factor of at least 15 to exposed areas.

• **Don't have X rays** any more frequently than is absolutely necessary. I no longer take routine annual chest films on my patients unless they're smokers, or have lung or heart disease. Some dentists are too enthusiastic about dental X rays. Make sure you really need them before acquiescing.

• **Such miscellaneous carcinogens** as asbestos, uranium, radon, benzene, and pesticides.

• **Long-term estrogen replacement therapy** predisposes women to cancer of the uterus (endometrial cancer), but adding progesterone nullifies that increased risk. However, estrogen may substantially raise the likelihood of breast cancer.

• **Chronic infection and inflammation** are responsible for about a third of the world's cancers. Liver cancer in particular, which is very common in Asia and Africa, is increasing in frequency in this country because of hepatitis B and C. (Hepatitis A, contracted from polluted food and water, almost always clears up in a few weeks after a brief illness and is not implicated in liver cancer.) The major villain is the hepatitis C virus, which is currently causing a worldwide epidemic. Both hepatitis B and C viruses are transmitted via infected blood (from transfusions, by sharing infected needles, and, in some 7 percent of cases, through sexual activity). Hepatitis B declares itself in no uncertain terms. After an incubation period of a few weeks, you begin to feel poorly, you lose your appetite, and you become jaundiced. A small percentage of cases go on to develop chronic liver disease, cirrhosis, and liver cancer. Hepatitis C is a much bigger problem because it's silent for so long. After the virus attacks the liver, it remains there, usually for decades, eating away at its cells without causing any symptoms. Unless you've had routine liver-function blood tests, you are not likely to suspect you're a carrier harboring hepatitis C. After many years, liver damage, including cirrhosis (scarring) and liver cancer, becomes evident. Unlike hepatitis A and B, there is as yet no vaccine against hepatitis C.

There are 170 million carriers of hepatitis C worldwide, 4 million of whom are in this country and have no idea they're at risk. (By contrast, only 1 million persons are infected with AIDS in the United States.) The majority with this disease contracted it from blood transfusions they received before 1990, when routine screening of blood for the virus first began. If you were given blood for any reason before 1990 or have at any time shared a needle with anyone or had sex with a stranger, I suggest that you have your blood checked for hepatitis C.

• **Schistosomiasis,** a parasitic disease widespread in Asia and Egypt and contracted from polluted water, can cause cancer of the colon and urinary bladder. Be careful where you swim when vacationing in those areas.

• **The human papilloma virus,** spread by sexual contact, is a major risk factor for cervical cancer.

• **Some drugs** used in the treatment of cancer, especially those that weaken the immune system, can actually cause another malignancy, such as leukemia, lymphoma, and sarcoma.

• **Air pollution,** especially indoors (where the concentration of pollutants is highest and where we spend 90 percent of our time), can cause cancer. The most important carcinogenic air pollutant is radon, a naturally occurring radioactive gas generated by the decay of trace amounts of radium in the earth's crust. Radon is believed to contribute to as many as 15,000 lung cancers a year in the United States, mostly among smokers (there is a synergistic effect between radon and tobacco). This gas enters houses primarily from the underlying soil. Recent research indicates that about one in twenty cases of lung cancer in the United Kingdom may be caused by residential radon, while in the United States it is estimated that 50,000 to 100,000 homes have radon levels twenty times the national average.

• **Water pollution** is not a great cancer risk. Chlorination of water, an extremely important and effective public-health measure that keeps teeth healthy, does produce some chlorinated by-products that can result in cancer in rodents, but nobody believes that this is an important cause of human cancer.

• *Helicobacter pylori,* the organism present in many peptic ulcers, is also associated with gastric cancer. A simple antibiotic regimen of one to two weeks eradicates

H. pylori, eliminating the possibility of it giving you stomach cancer.

Cancer prevention means controlling as many of these risk factors as possible and having regular checkups for its early detection.

Detecting Cancer

A checkup is a fishing expedition for the earliest evidence of any silent disease or disorder, including cancer. The focus of the routine physical depends on your age, vulnerability, and sex. If you have specific symptoms, fears, or susceptibility, your doctor will perform a targeted exam. But don't wait until you're sick. Get your physical while you're still healthy.

During a general checkup, your doctor should obtain a detailed medical history so that he or she can pay special attention to areas of potential disease. Most doctors spend so little time with their patients these days, especially the presumably healthy ones, that instead of asking you these questions face to face, they give you a printed form to answer. Don't gloss over it. Think carefully about each question; it may remind you of something you've forgotten to tell the doctor or didn't think was important. And be sure to discuss any query to which you answered yes.

A careful, total body physical exam is extremely important. Beware of any doctor who examines you while you're partially dressed; you should be wearing nothing so that every part of your body is visible. No exam is complete without an examination of all your lymph glands—in the neck, the armpit, and the groin—as well as a digital evaluation of the rectum and, in women, a pelvic exam too.

After the physical, you should have your urine checked for evidence of infection, blood, and abnormal proteins; your stool should be analyzed for the presence of blood (it's not always visible to the naked eye); and your blood should be drawn for a spectrum of tests. Recent government legislation (which I opposed without success when I served on the Practicing Physicians' Advisory Council to the Secretary of Health) prohibits Medicare from reimbursing you for screening blood tests if you have no specific complaints. This is a big blow to preventive medicine. Our lawmakers apparently have yet to realize that early diagnosis and treatment cost much less than waiting for trouble to appear. Over the years, I have diagnosed a host of unexpected abnormalities: cancer (from the chemical detection of blood in the stool); thyroid underfunction (from a routine blood test in patients who believed they were simply "tired"); diabetes (from urine or blood of patients who never suspected that their sugar was elevated); kidney trouble; liver disease; abnormal cholesterol and other blood-fat levels; tumors of the parathyroid gland (when the only abnormality was a high calcium level in the blood); and hepatitis C. If you're in the Medicare age group, or if you're younger and your insurance carrier or managed-care company won't pay for routine blood tests, then arrange with your doctor so that he or she performs them anyway.

In order to detect early cancer, certain tests should routinely be done at varying intervals, not necessarily annually, depending on your age, sex, and the type of cancer (or other disease) to which you are especially susceptible. Although X rays of the upper gastrointestinal tract and barium enemas are still widely used, newer techniques are often preferred when there is a suspicious finding. For example, the *CT scan* is a special procedure in which a computer is hooked up to an X-ray machine and a series of detailed pictures is taken at different levels or "cuts" of the tissue being examined. This provides an in-depth analysis of a particular region of the body, such as the chest or the abdomen. *Endoscopy* allows the doctor to view the interior of the body through a thin tube with a light and a little snare at its end. (Such an exam is named for the organ being studied: A colonoscopy looks inside the colon; gastroscopy views the stomach; and bronchoscopy visualizes the respiratory system.) Looking directly at these tissues makes it possible to remove a polyp or to snip a piece off any suspicious tissue that is present and send it to the lab for analysis. The pathologist stains the cells, looks at them under the microscope, and can tell whether they're cancerous, and, if so, whether they are likely to grow slowly or quickly.

Radionuclear scanning is a noninvasive procedure in which you are given a mildly radioactive substance orally or by injection. A scanner measures the radioactivity level of the area or organ being evaluated and prints a picture of it on paper or film. The radioactive uptake pattern reveals the presence of growths and other abnormalities in the target tissue.

Ultrasound is a useful diagnostic procedure that is usually done to clarify a suspicious finding in the physical exam. High-frequency sound waves that cannot be heard by humans are directed toward the organ in question. Their "echo" bounces back to produce a picture called a sonogram, which appears on a monitor, and is then printed on paper for a permanent record. Sonograms are especially valuable in the diagnosis of heart disease. However, they also reveal cancers in the abdomen that the doctor cannot feel, for example, in the pancreas, gallbladder, or liver.

Magnetic resonance imaging (MRI) involves the use of a powerful magnet linked to a computer that gives detailed pictures of various areas of the body. There is no radiation involved; the derived information is viewed on a monitor, and then printed out. With the exception of endoscopy, the MRI probably yields more information about cancer than any of the other diagnostic procedures described above.

Cancer-Focused Exams

On what aspects of the checkup should the doctor concentrate when looking for cancer? Listed below are some of the cancer-focused exams that you should have on a regular basis in order to detect the disease at an early stage.

• **Breast Cancer:** Women over the age of sixty-five

who are at greatest risk for breast cancer (there is more detailed information on this subject at the end of this chapter) should take the following three steps to ensure its early detection:

1. A mammogram. Properly done and carefully interpreted, this X-ray procedure identifies a breast tumor as early as two years before it can be felt.
2. Self-examination of your own breasts every month. Learn the right way to do it either from your doctor or by phoning the National Cancer Institute at 1-800-422-6237 (1-800-4-CANCER). They'll send you a free booklet.
3. A breast exam by your doctor during your regular health checkup or at least every year.

• **Uterine and cervical cancer:** As a woman grows older, her risk of cancer of the uterus and cervix increases. Some women stop seeing their gynecologist after menopause because they think that since their periods have ended, there are no more potential "female" problems. That's a mistake. Someone—a gynecologist or your family doctor—should do a pelvic exam and Pap test once a year regardless of how old you are. Although some doctors believe that if you've had a normal Pap test for three consecutive years after menopause, you may skip it, I still recommend that it be done annually.

• **Cancer of the colon and rectum** are also more common in older persons. Three tests can detect this malignancy:

1. The guaiac stool test (also called the fecal, or stool, occult test, or hemoccult test) reveals the presence of traces of blood in the stool not visible to the naked eye. You can do this one yourself with a kit available at all pharmacies. It comes with explicit instructions. A chemical is added to the specimen, and a change in color indicates the presence of blood.

2. An annual rectal exam, in which the doctor feels for any bumps or irregular areas of the rectum. (This is a must at every regular checkup. Insist on it.)

3. Colonoscopy every three to five years beginning at age fifty. A long thin tube is inserted via the rectum and threaded the entire length of the colon. (Sigmoidoscopy is a similar procedure, but the instrument doesn't reach nearly as far.) This allows the doctor to inspect the lining of the bowel and detect any polyps or growths. You'd never suspect it from my photograph, but I am older than fifty, and, until recently, never had a colonoscopy despite a family history of colon cancer. ("Do as I say, not as I do.") Why not? Because I was afraid of the discomfort and pain. Finally, after a trip to India, I developed some symptoms that left me no choice. My doctor (and, more important, my wife) insisted that I have the colonoscopy. I swear there's absolutely nothing to it! The doctor gives you some sedatives that leave you groggy but awake—I felt absolutely nothing. So if you've been putting off having your colonoscopy done because you're afraid, call your doctor and set it up. You won't feel it—or regret it. (P.S.: My test was normal.)

• **Prostate cancer** is the most common malignancy among American men, 80 percent of whom are sixty-five and older. (Unlike skin cancer, you can't look for this one yourself.) This malignancy is discussed in detail later in this chapter.

• **Skin cancer:** Your doctor should inspect your skin carefully in the course of every routine physical exam. That's not done often enough. Some "blemishes" can be so tricky that I refer my own patients to a dermatologist once a year to have their entire body surface checked for malignant or premalignant lesions. You can improve the chances of finding one early in the game by inspecting your skin yourself. (I admit that the back presents a problem.) Look for and report anything that's suspicious to you, especially if it's changed in size, texture, color, its borders have become irregular, or is a sore that doesn't heal.

Look specifically for moles or pigmented spots on the skin. (Doctors call them nevi.) They first appear as small, flat, tan or brown spots that slowly become raised. In time, they can flatten again, become flesh-colored, and disappear. Nevi are specific cells in the skin (melanocytes) that have heaped up in a cluster instead of spreading out evenly. (Melanocytes give the skin its natural color. When you sit in the sun, your melanocytes produce more pigment, darkening and tanning the skin.) Most people normally have anywhere from ten to forty nevi, and develop new ones from time to time until approximately age forty. At least one of every ten of them is dysplastic, an unusual-looking or atypical mole different from the rest. Dysplastic nevi are more likely than the others to develop into a melanoma. (However, most don't.) Any skin lesion that's the least bit suspicious looking should be biopsied. That's the only way to be sure it isn't malignant.

You should check your mouth at regular intervals, and so should your doctor and dentist. Look for changes in the color of your lips and tongue. Then open wide ("Ahh" is optional) and inspect the inner cheeks; search everywhere for scabs, cracks, sores, white patches, swelling, or bleeding. Report what you find to your doctor.

Skin cancer is the most common tumor in this country, in both men and women. Fortunately, most skin cancers, such as the basal or squamous cell types, are localized, easily removable, and rarely threaten life. However, a malignant melanoma is potentially fatal and must be removed early—before it spreads throughout the body. This cancer is caused by exposure to ultraviolet radiation from the sun, sunlamps, and tanning booths. People at greatest risk for melanomas are those who've already had one, who have close relatives with them, who were badly sunburned as children or teenagers, or whose skin is fair and burns or freckles easily. The incidence of malignant melanoma rose almost 80 percent between 1973 and 1988, and it continues to do so—more than any other cancer.

Symptoms Suspicious of Cancer

Here are some important body signals to follow up without fail:

• **Any change in bowel habits.** If you've always enjoyed normal bowel movements but suddenly develop constipation that continues for two weeks or more, especially if it's accompanied by intermittent attacks of diarrhea, let your doctor know. Cancer of the bowel often presents itself in this way. Blood in the stool, even if you would like to attribute it to your hemorrhoids (why aren't they called "asteroids"?), should also be checked out because hemorrhoids can coexist with more serious colon problems. Finally, if your normally bulky stool has become thin and ribbonlike, the reduced caliber may be due to a growth that's narrowing a portion of the colon.

• **An open sore** or a persistent rash that does not clear up may reflect skin cancer.

• **Blood or discharge** from any body orifice—vomited, coughed up, in the urine, from the vagina, or in the stool—must be explained.

• **Show your doctor any persistent bump or lump** anywhere you find it—in the breast, on the skin, in the testicle, under your arms, in your neck, your groin, or in your abdomen.

• **Pain in your stomach,** either when you're hungry or after you eat, indigestion, or difficulty swallowing, may all be important danger signals.

- **A chronic, nagging cough,** with or without sputum and especially (but not necessarily) accompanied by any amount of blood, however small, is an ominous sign—especially in smokers. So is persistent hoarseness.

- **A low-grade fever** without an obvious cause (doctors call it FUO—fever of unknown origin) that continues for longer than a week or two warrants a visit to your doctor. It may be due to something as innocuous as an infection behind a tooth or an allergic response to some medication you're taking, but it may also reflect a serious process such as a diseased heart valve, an abscess somewhere in the body—or a hidden malignancy.

- **If you're losing weight** for no apparent reason, you should have a thorough checkup. The problem may be some medication you're taking (a notorious culprit is digitalis, widely used for treating various heart conditions), an overactive thyroid, an undiagnosed infection—or, again, a hidden cancer.

Do not ignore any of these warning signs simply because they are not causing you any pain—at the moment. Cancers often don't hurt in the early stages.

If You Have Cancer

If you're told you have cancer, either as a result of a routine checkup or in the course of having some symptom evaluated, all is not lost. Many malignancies can either be cured or controlled for years, especially if they are detected and treated early enough. There are millions of people who had colon, breast, stomach, prostate, uterine, skin, and other cancers who are now leading active, normal lives.

If you have cancer, consider getting a second opinion, both to confirm the diagnosis and to make sure that the treatment plan suggested is the best one available. Some insurance companies require such a consultation; others leave it up to you but will pay for it. You can either ask your doctor to recommend a specialist or you can call the National Cancer Institute at 1-800-4-CANCER (1-800-422-6237). They'll refer you to the closest cancer treatment center and provide you with a list of doctors who have the most experience in your particular problem.

Ask your doctor the following key questions:

- What is the exact diagnosis?
- What is the stage of disease?
- What are my treatment choices; which one do you recommend and why?
- What are the risks, possible side effects, and chances of success of each treatment?
- What will be the duration of the treatment? How will it affect my normal activities?
- How much is it likely to cost? (Always check with your insurance carrier to see whether they will cover the recommended treatment.)
- Are there any clinical trials of a new treatment in which I should be enrolled if the therapy for my particular cancer is not usually successful?

Treating Cancer

The treatment of cancer depends on the type, the organ affected, whether it is localized or has spread, and your general state of health (some therapies may be too taxing for someone who is frail).

Wherever possible, cancer should be removed *surgically*. Unfortunately, this is not always possible. Nearby lymph nodes are also excised to see if the tumor has spread to them.

Radiation therapy may be an option, either when surgery is not feasible or when the surgeon isn't able to remove the tumor completely. However, it may be the first choice when the cancer is localized and its cells are radiosensitive, as, for example, in prostate cancer. The high-energy rays destroy the cancer cells, or damage them so that they stop growing and dividing. Radiation is delivered either externally from a machine or internally from an implant, in which case a small radioactive container is placed directly into or near the tumor. (Some patients with prostate cancer receive both internal and external radiation.) External radiation is usually administered on an outpatient basis five days a week for several weeks. It doesn't leave you radioactive; you can't spread the rays to those near you. Internal radiation therapy, on the other hand, requires an operation in order to implant the radioactive receptacle. Implants may be permanent or removed after a certain period of time.

Chemotherapy refers to the administration of medication, sometimes orally, but more commonly by injection into a vein or muscle. Chemotherapy slows down the progression of the disease but does not usually cure the cancer. It's a systemic treatment that reaches every organ of the body through the bloodstream. Unfortunately, many of these agents are toxic and also attack normal tissues. When intravenous chemotherapy is given over a period of time, the doctor will often administer it through a catheter (a thin, flexible tube) inserted into a large vein in the chest. This saves sticking you repeatedly, and reduces the risk of some of these powerful substances leaking out of the vein and destroying surrounding tissues. Chemotherapy is usually given in cycles, at an outpatient clinic of a hospital, at the doctor's office, or at home. But if you're fragile to begin with, and are receiving potent drugs with side effects that need special attention, you may be admitted to the hospital for a few days.

Cancers of organs such as the prostate, breast, and ovary that secrete hormones or are dependent on them are usually surgically removed and/or treated with *hormones*. Like chemotherapy, hormones affect the entire body.

Immunotherapy therapy, a more recent approach to the treatment of cancer, holds considerable promise. It utilizes the body's immune system to fight the cancer and/or to protect it from some of the side effects of other treatments. Tumor cells from the patient are inactivated and then injected into a laboratory animal, where they stimulate the production of specific antibodies to the cancer. These antibodies are then removed from the animal and injected into the patient, in whom they make a beeline directly for the tumor, attacking it and sparing healthy tissue. These monoclonal (or sometimes polyclonal) anti-bodies can also be attached to chemotherapy drugs and other antitumor agents, which selectively search out the tumor. An exciting recent advance in this field is her-ceptin, a laboratory-designed monoclonal antibody. When given to women with breast cancer who have the HER2 gene (present in 30 percent of breast cancers), this agent targets and destroys the protein that makes the can-cer grow.

Biological therapy is also relatively new. Patients are given various natural substances such as interferon, inter-leukin 2, and several types of colony-stimulating factors, all of which enhance the body's own defenses.

New advances in the prevention and treatment of can-cer are reported virtually every week. A novel approach currently being evaluated is the use of *anti-angiogenic agents* that destroy the blood supply of the tumor instead of attacking it directly. The tumors shrivel and die when deprived of their nourishment—at least in mice. These drugs are now being evaluated in humans. Initial reports were not promising at the time of writing, but that may change. In one study of twenty-four patients with various types of cancer, only one, a man with kidney cancer, showed significant shrinkage of his tumor after receiving one of these agents—the tumor decreased by 39 percent. In another study of thirty-three patients with advanced kidney cancer, only one showed partial shrinkage of the tumor. However, in four others, who continued the treat-ment for a full year, the cancer did not spread.

There has been an explosion of knowledge in the field

of *gene therapy*. Several genes responsible for cancer of the breast, ovary, lung, and other organs have already been identified. I believe it's just a matter of time before their mutations can be prevented, or possibly reversed.

Nutrition often poses a problem in cancer patients, especially those with extensive or advanced disease, many of whom develop an aversion to food. Most conventional physicians encourage them to eat as much as they can. However, some alternative practitioners recommend starving the cancer. I have never seen any real effect on survival from either of these courses of action. However, I favor the "let them eat" philosophy because, in my experience, the more cancer patients eat, the better they feel, the more energy they have, and the more capable they are of handling the side effects of treatment.

The Side Effects of Cancer Treatment

Most cancer therapy produces a range of side effects that varies from life-threatening to merely making you feel miserable. Surgery, for example, not only cures, it also kills. Someone who is old and sick, whether from the cancer alone or also from another serious disease, may be a high risk for a major operation. This puts the surgeon and the cancer patient between a rock and a hard place, especially when surgery offers the only chance of a cure. Even if you survive the operation, it takes time to recover fully from the anesthesia, the blood loss, and the trauma. Expect to feel tired and weak, at least for a little while.

Given their focus on saving money (and under pressure from the government and insurance companies to do so), the hospital may want to send you home before you've fully recovered. If you're too weak to take care of yourself properly at home, you have the right to refuse to leave. Most hospitals will back down (especially if you tell them you've got a good lawyer).

Whether or not radiation therapy knocks the stuffing out of you depends on the dose you receive and the part of the body being treated. For example, radiating a malignancy in the head and neck, or the tongue, can make your teeth fall out and so inflame the tissues of the mouth and throat that eating and swallowing are difficult and painful. The rays can also hurt the bone marrow, reducing its production of white blood cells that protect the body against infection. Generally speaking, however, the most common adverse effects of radiation are fatigue, rash, redness in the treated area, and loss of appetite. Most of these side effects can be prevented or controlled with the newer equipment that pinpoints the target tissue with greater accuracy and reduces the risk of overdosing.

Chemotherapy causes the most troublesome side effects because most of the drugs used also damage healthy cells. It can affect the bone marrow so that it makes fewer white blood cells (that fight infection), platelets (responsible for normal clotting), and red blood cells (that carry oxygen). As a result, you don't resist infections nearly as well, you bruise and bleed more easily, and you're tired because you're anemic. There are now medications that can stimulate a damaged marrow to make enough white cells and red cells to keep you going. However, if the drug (or radiation) has hurt the bone marrow badly enough, you may require a total marrow transplant or replacement of just the specific tissue that forms blood cells (peripheral stem cell support).

Chemotherapy can also affect the digestive tract and cause nausea, vomiting, and sores in the mouth. Acupuncture can minimize some of these effects, as does marijuana (don't tell the cops I told you). Hair loss is a major concern too, especially in women. The hair either thins out or is lost throughout the body (alopecia) for the duration of the therapy, which may be many months. However, hair usually begins to grow back after the treatment is completed. Chemotherapy also impairs fertility in both sexes, either temporarily or permanently.

Hormone therapy can also cause side effects. Women may develop swelling, weight gain, hot flashes, and vaginal dryness, and become infertile. In men with prostate cancer, the antitestosterone drugs that control the spread of their tumor also invariably result in temporary or permanent impotence, loss of sexual desire, and loss of fertility. Nausea and vomiting can occur in both sexes.

The side effects of biological therapy and immunotherapy depend on the specific agents being used. Interferon, for example, causes flu-like symptoms that are often severe: chills, fever, muscle aches, weakness, nausea, loss of appetite, vomiting, and diarrhea. Some patients also develop a rash and bleeding. However, these symptoms are usually transient, and they will clear up after the treatment is completed.

PROSTATE CANCER AND BREAST CANCER

Since cancer of the breast and prostate are so common and exact such a toll in the aging population, I have chosen to discuss their prevention and treatment separately.

Prostate Cancer

Cancer of the prostate is the second biggest cancer killer of men in this country (after lung cancer) and their most common nonskin malignancy; there are approximately 200,000 new cases diagnosed every year, and more than 40,000 deaths. Unlike some other forms of cancer, prostate cancer does not usually give symptoms in its early and curable stage. However, once the cancer spreads, it causes pain in the organ it has attacked. This malignancy is most likely to affect bone, and it is a common cause of sudden, nonarthritic, unexplained pain in the spine.

DIAGNOSING PROSTATE CANCER

Since early cancer of the prostate is usually silent, you've got to look for it. Eighty percent of cases occur after the age of sixty-five, but I start screening all my male patients at age fifty. For some reason, African-American males are 50 percent more likely to have prostate cancer than are white Americans, so it's extremely important that they first be tested for it early (age forty-five), and annually thereafter.

Both your doctor's gloved finger and your blood are usually required to diagnose prostate cancer. In many cases, but not always (which is why blood tests are needed), the doctor will feel a hard, irregular, lumpy, cancerous gland (instead of the soft, smooth consistency of the normal prostate). It may or may not be enlarged. Although some have questioned the cost-effectiveness of the PSA (prostate specific antigen) test, in which the blood level of this protein made only by the prostate is measured, it should always be done along with the digital rectal exam. PSA readings are increased in men with benign prostatic hypertrophy and infections of the prostate gland as well as in cancer patients, but every high PSA should be considered cancer until proven otherwise. Most doctors accept a PSA range from 1 to 4 (nanograms) as normal. However, if your PSA has always remained between 1 and 2 and is now close to 4, the prostate should be further evaluated. The transrectal ultrasound test should be done when there is any doubt about the size or consistency of the prostate gland, or when the PSA is questionable. An instrument inserted into the rectum directs sound waves to the prostate; their echo pattern is converted by a computer into a picture that is studied for any irregularity. Suspicious findings usually require a biopsy of the gland—a simple procedure in which a needle is inserted into the gland to obtain

some of its tissue, which is then studied under the microscope for the presence of cancerous cells.

Recently, doctors have also been using a refinement of
the PSA, in which its "free fraction" (the part of the PSA
protein that is unattached) is measured too. When the free
PSA is less than 25 percent of the total, the likelihood of
cancer is high. This test has reduced the need to perform
a needle biopsy in borderline cases. A biopsy tells us if
cancer is present and whether it is aggressive or slow-
growing. This, together with the age and general health of
the patient, helps determine what the treatment should be.

TREATING PROSTATE CANCER

Diagnosing prostate cancer is the easy part; how best to
treat it presents more of a problem. The decision depends
on the size of the tumor, its stage (whether or not it has
spread beyond the confines of the prostate gland), the activity of the cells (whether they are fairly dormant or are
multiplying rapidly), your age (the older you are, the less
aggressive the treatment should be), and, as important as
any other consideration, your lifestyle and your personal
preferences.

The main problem in deciding what treatment to have
arises when the cancer is small and in its early stages.
Following are some of your options.

You can wait it out. If you're in your seventies or eighties and the cancer is small and not aggressive, chances
are you will outlive it. Many doctors and older patients,

especially if they have any other serious illness, prefer to follow this "living with it" course rather than to have surgery or radiation—the other two major options. (It takes a certain mind-set to be able to "live with a cancer," but in Europe, particularly Sweden, this is how such tumors are usually managed.) If you decide on this course, you will need to see your urologist at frequent and regular intervals to make sure the cancer is quiescent. I have followed many such patients for years and years, and their tumors have not flared up or spread.

If you're young—say under seventy—and in good health, your best bet is to remove the cancer and surrounding tissues surgically (called a *radical prostatectomy*). This cannot always be done if the tumor is very large, and certainly not if it's already spread. The advantages of surgery are that, when successful, the cancer is out and you're done with it; the downside is the side effects. In the past, this operation always resulted in impotence because the nerves alongside the prostate that control erection were removed or otherwise damaged during the procedure. With the "nerve-sparing" technique devised by Dr. Patrick Walsh at Johns Hopkins (and now performed virtually everywhere), 40 to 70 percent of men retain the ability to have an erection. However, the threat of impotence persists. (There are many ways to treat this complication, the newest of which is Viagra.) Incontinence, the inability to hold the urine, is another postoperative complication. Although most men regain urinary control after a few weeks, some do not. Finally, a radical prostatectomy is not a trivial operation, and, as is true for any surgery, you may not be able to tolerate the anesthesia; you may lose blood and require transfusions; you may develop blood clots, infection, or pneumonia; or even sustain a heart attack if your cardiac status was impaired to begin with. So if you decide to go this route, get a good checkup first. The great majority of properly selected patients do well, and the long-term results are good, too.

Now, if the tumor is still localized but needs to be treated and you prefer not to have an operation, or if the cancer is inoperable, you can have *radiation therapy;* high-energy rays kill the cancer cells and shrink the tumor. This is the simplest of all the treatments. When properly done, the ten-year survival rate and the side effects are comparable to those of surgery. If you choose radiation, make sure you receive your treatment from a specialist skilled in radiation of the prostate.

There are two kinds of radiation treatment for prostate cancer, and they're sometimes given together. External radiation is the more widely used of the two. I insist that all my patients get the three-dimensional conformal external radiation rather than the standard therapy. This is a more powerful treatment in which a computer pinpoints multiple X-ray beams directly to the cancer, with very little spillover to nearby tissues or organs. This approach makes it possible to deliver more radiation with less inflammation, diarrhea, impotence, and incontinence than standard radiation. You'll have to go to the clinic for about fifteen minutes once a day, five days a week, for six or seven weeks.

Radiation can also be given internally by the implantation of radioactive pellets directly into and around the cancerous prostate, guided by ultrasound. This process is called *brachytherapy*. It involves a one- to two-hour operation under general or regional anesthesia. You can have either high-energy pellets that deliver a large dose of radiation and are removed after a few days or, more commonly, low-energy pellets that are permanently implanted. If you choose internal radiation, don't worry; you won't be radioactive to others. The key to the success of this form of therapy is the accurate positioning of the pellets, something that requires skill and experience. Properly done, side effects are minimal. Many cancer centers are combining external and internal radiation in suitable subjects.

If the cancer has spread, your options are fairly limited. At this stage, treatment is directed at controlling your pain and trying to slow down the further dissemination of the malignancy. You will be offered direct *radiation* to the area, usually to bones that are now harboring the tumor, and you will also be given *antitestosterone hormones,* since prostate cancer is dependent to some extent on this male hormone. Before the discovery of these hormone medications (Lupron or Zolodex, given by injection every one or three months and often supplemented by daily oral doses), the only way to cut down testosterone production was to remove the testes surgically. This is now done much less often, for obvious reasons. Hormone therapy usually has feminizing effects such as loss of libido and enlargement of the breasts, and it often becomes less effective after two or three years.

The foregoing represents the conventional or establishment view on the diagnosis and treatment of prostate cancer, a position with which I happen to agree. However, you should know that a growing number of urologists disagree. In their opinion, the PSA test should not be done because only 30 percent of men with abnormal readings turn out to have prostate cancer. Such "false-positive" results lead to unnecessary invasive tsting, not to mention the anxiety of being told one may have cancer. About 3 percent of men who really do have cancer have normal PSA results. Some urologists also believe that the great majority of prostate cancers are so slow growing that most men outlive them, and die of other causes. They recommend "watchful waiting" of all such malignancies.

Many of these arguments are true, and pose a moral and philosophical dilemma to doctors and patients alike. My problem with this nihilistic position is that no one can predict how a given prostate cancer will behave. Most of my patients and I are unwilling to play Russian roulette with their lives. They want to know whether or not they have cancer, and if they do, they almost always want it treated, regardless of the statistics. However, you should base your own decision about testing for and treating prostate cancer with your own doctor.

On the horizon are newer techniques that will stimulate the immune system and keep the cancer under control. Specific antibodies to the prostate cancer cells are injected, and then ideally make a beeline for the malignant tissue.

Prevention is the best cure. Although there's no guarantee, I think you can reduce your risk of developing prostate cancer with a diet that's low in fat and rich in vegetables, tomatoes (with their high concentration of lycopenes), whole grains, fruits, and soy. Many doctors believe such a diet is the reason this disease is less common in Asia than in the West. When Chinese and Japanese men leave their homeland, move here, abandon their old eating habits, and adopt ours, the incidence of prostate cancer among them is as high as yours and mine. Recent research also suggests that men with higher blood levels of selenium (a trace metal found in many foods) have a lower incidence of prostate cancer than do those with lower levels. It's too early to advise you to take selenium supplements for this purpose, but keep your eyes peeled for more definitive trials in the future. I also believe that taking testosterone to try to improve your libido or sexual performance when you're not deficient in it may increase the risk of prostate cancer. However, this theory has not been proved.

Breast Cancer

One woman in eight will develop breast cancer in her lifetime (it used to be one in fourteen back in 1960), making it the most common cancer among females in this country. More than 200,000 new cases are diagnosed each year, and there are 45,000 deaths. Looked at another way, one new case of breast cancer is diagnosed every three minutes, and it kills someone every twelve minutes. It is the leading cause of cancer deaths among African Americans, and is the number-one killer among *all* women between forty and fifty-five years of age.

The risk of breast cancer increases as you get older, and two-thirds of all cases occur after the age of fifty. But there are risk factors other than age, including a strong family history. However, most women with breast cancer don't have predictable risk factors, and that means that you have to keep looking for it throughout your adult life, regardless of whether or not you are statistically vulnerable. To do so, you must learn how to examine your breasts yourself and then do it regularly once a month. (Women find many more breast abnormalities than their doctors do.) An annual screening mammogram after age forty is important because breast cancer can be cured if caught in time (and, as noted earlier, a mammogram can pick it up two years before any lump can be felt). The five-year survival rate for localized breast cancer is a whopping 93 percent! Strangely enough, despite their worry about this disease, only a minority of women examine their breasts regularly, and less than one-third have an annual mammogram.

RISK FACTORS FOR BREAST CANCER

- **A family history of breast cancer** (mothers, sisters, aunts) is important. Although you can't change it, it can alert you to your vulnerability. If the familial incidence is high—if your mother and two sisters all had breast and/or ovarian cancers, especially prior to menopause—you may want to discuss with your doctor whether you should be tested for the genes (BrCa1, BrCa2, P53) that are markers of susceptibility. If the results are positive, you should consider prophylactic tamoxifen or raloxifene (see below), or even a prophylactic mastectomy. The latter substantially reduces the risk of breast cancer, although it's not a guarantee of protection since some breast tissue usually remains behind.

• **As discussed above, several other risk factors** such as smoking, alcohol, weight gain, and a diet rich in fat and light on fruits and vegetables may contribute to breast cancer.

• **The risk of breast cancer is greater, too, if you started menstruating** before the age of twelve and your menopause did not take place until age fifty-five. That's because of your longer exposure to estrogen. By the same token, if your ovaries were surgically removed for whatever reason before age forty or forty-five, your chances of getting breast cancer are reduced because of your shorter exposure to this hormonal stimulation.

• **Never having had children,** or giving birth for the first time after the age of thirty, raises the risk of breast cancer. That's one of the reasons nuns have a disproportionately high rate of breast cancer. So if you're going to have babies, do so when you're young. After you have your baby, remember that breast-feeding reduces the incidence of breast cancer, too.

• **Women whose breasts are large and heavy** are at higher risk of breast cancer, presumably because small, early tumors are harder to detect in such cases and so treatment is delayed. It's especially important for such women to have regular mammograms.

• **Being overweight and relatively tall** appears to raise the risk of breast cancer. (Rates of breast cancer have apparently gone up in countries where adult height has increased, as for example, in Japan, where women are taller than they used to be.) However, this apparent adverse influence of height and weight may simply reflect the consequences of a high-fat diet.

• **If you've had cancer of the uterus, ovary, or colon,** you're at twice the risk of getting breast cancer—and vice versa.

• **Estrogen** has been implicated as a cause of breast cancer, which is one reason that so many women avoid it. My own feeling is that where there's smoke, there's fire, and that estrogen probably does increase the risk somewhat. However, its other benefits (a sense of well-being, reduced incidence of osteoporosis, fewer heart attacks and strokes, and less severe Alzheimer's) so outweigh the risks that I recommend estrogen to most of my postmenopausal patients. However, they and I are then much more careful about monitoring the breasts. Although the addition of progesterone does reduce the risk of endometrial (uterine) cancer posed by taking estrogen alone, giving it along with the estrogen may increase the risk of developing breast cancer.

PREVENTING BREAST CANCER

Prophylactic tamoxifen reduces the risk of breast cancer by as much as 45 percent in high-risk females and those over the age of sixty. This observation has generated an ongoing debate as to whether these women should take this drug. Since the study which documented this beneficial effect ran for only four years, we can't be sure that taking tamoxifen for longer than that won't actually enhance the risk of cancer later on, as it seems to do when given for more than five years as prophylaxis after breast-cancer treatment. Also, as mentioned below, tamoxifen is associated with a higher risk of blood clotting, embolism to the lungs, and cancer of the uterus. However, these complications are relatively infrequent by comparison to the incidence of breast cancer, and they can all be avoided and even successfully treated if such patients are carefully monitored.

The bottom line? It seems to me that any woman at high risk for breast cancer, especially after the age of fifty, should seriously consider taking tamoxifen. At the time of writing, raloxifene (marketed as Evista in the United States), which is currently approved for the prevention and treatment of osteoporosis, is now being investigated for its breast-cancer-prevention potential. Initial reports are very promising. And, as is the case with many other cancers and diseases, exercise and diet are very important preventatives. Exercise appears to lower the risk of breast cancer in young women by influencing estrogen levels.

A diet low in fat and high in vegetable intake is also help-ful. In particular, foods such as soybeans contain weakly es-trogenic substances that compete with more potent natural estrogens and so may reduce the risk of breast cancer.

DIAGNOSING BREAST CANCER

Supposing you find what appears to be a lump in your breast (cancerous lumps are generally hard, painless, and the skin covering them may be dimpled, like the rind of an orange) or a mammogram is said to be "suspicious." Where do you go from here? First, keep your cool. Eighty percent of these lumps turn out to be benign, and half the biopsies done because of questionable mammograms are normal. But you can't count on these statistics. Regardless of the presence or absence of any risk factors, or what you or your doctor *think* the lump or mammogram may mean, it must be investigated. Do not make such a life-and-death decision on the basis of how the lump looks, its size, and what it feels like. *You must have a tissue diagnosis.* That means your doctor must obtain a sample of the tissue from the lump and look at it under a microscope. Depending on the size of the mass and its location in the breast, that may re-quire either an open biopsy (an incision is made and a piece of the tissue is removed), or a fine needle aspiration (a nee-dle is inserted into the tumor and some of its contents are sucked up). The open biopsy, though invasive, is usually more accurate, but a "hit" with a fine needle aspiration is also reliable.

TREATING BREAST CANCER

There are several standard approaches to the treatment of breast cancer. The *lumpectomy* has become more popular because of the limited surgery involved. In this procedure, the tumor, along with any surrounding cancerous tissue as well as a border of healthy tissue surrounding the cancer, are removed. However, this procedure can only be done safely if the tumor is a single one; if other parts of the breast, especially the nipple, are not involved; and the tumor is less than two inches across. Lumpectomy should be followed by radiation to the breast given for two minutes daily for five weeks. Chemotherapy is sometimes also recommended to "take care" of any cancer cells elsewhere in the body. The most recent long-term follow-up studies suggest that lumpectomy, in properly selected women, is as effective as a mastectomy.

The *simple mastectomy,* in which the entire breast is removed, is usually reserved for intraductal cancers. These are not suitable for lumpectomy, and do not require the more extensive modified radical procedure.

In the *skin-sparing mastectomy,* the breast surgeon and a plastic surgeon work together to conserve as much skin from the healthy portion of the breast as possible. They use it to rebuild the breast using either the patient's own tissues or saline-filled implants. In this operation, the same amount of breast tissue is removed as during a simple mastectomy, but the outer skin is left intact. This procedure is not done in someone with recurrent breast cancer, after a lumpectomy and radiation, or in women whose cancers are located close to the skin.

A *modified radical mastectomy*, in which the entire breast and the glands in the armpit are removed, is another surgical option.

Surgery is only the first step in the therapy of breast cancer. After the tissue is removed, it is analyzed to see whether its cells take up or "bind" with female hormones. The cancer is then designated as either "receptor positive" or "receptor negative." If it's positive, your doctor should prescribe the anti-estrogen drug tamoxifen for five years, but no longer. This substantially improves the long-term outlook in most cases, and reduces the chances of a new cancer developing in the other breast. Tamoxifen does other good things, too: It lowers cholesterol and has a positive effect on osteoporosis. However, its downside is important: weight gain, a tendency for the blood to clot in the veins and cause a pulmonary embolism, and, most important, a greater risk of uterine cancer. (Of course, the latter complication does not occur if you've previously had a hysterectomy.) So discuss the pros and cons of tamoxifen with your doctor. In the great majority of cases, the pluses outweigh the minuses. But if you take it, you will need to have careful, ongoing surveillance.

If your tumor is receptor negative or if the cancer has spread to the lymph glands under your arm, you'll need *chemotherapy*. Currently, the most effective regimen consists of four drugs—Cytoxan (cyclophosphamide), Rheumatrex (methotrexate), Adriamycin (doxorubicin), and 5-fluorouracil. Your oncologist will decide how long you should continue them. These drugs cause side effects that range from hair loss to nausea and cardiac damage, but they're worth enduring to reap their long-term benefits. Taxol, made from the bark of the yew tree, is also effective in the treatment of early-stage breast cancer when it's combined with chemotherapy. It prolongs survival in 26 percent of cases, and reduces the risk of recurrence by 22 percent.

While cancer remains a terrifying disease, there is much that can be done to prevent and treat it. I'm optimistic that the battle will be won, that one day soon scientists will either "conquer" cancer or come up with some answers that will significantly lower its death toll.

The table below lists the main symptoms of some common cancers and how they're usually treated.

TYPE OF CANCER	STAGE	SYMPTOM	RECOMMENDED TREATMENT
Lung Cancer	Early	Persistent cough	Surgery, radiation therapy
	Late	Cough with blood	Chemotherapy + radiation therapy
Breast Cancer	Early	Breast lump	Surgery, radiation therapy
	Late	Breast lump; enlarged glands in armpit; spread to bones, brain, and other organs	Chemotherapy

Head and Neck Cancer	Early	Swelling in affected area	Surgery + radiation therapy
	Late	Same	Chemotherapy
Gastric Cancer	Early	Abdominal pain after eating	Surgery
	Late	Diffuse abdominal pain	Chemotherapy
Esophageal Cancer	Early	Difficulty swallowing	Surgery
	Late	Same	Chemotherapy, radiation therapy
Renal Cancer	Early	Blood in urine, back pain	Surgery
	Late	Same	Immunotherapy, chemotherapy
Melanoma	Early	Suspicious-looking mole	Surgery
	Late	Evidence of spread to other organs	Immunotherapy, chemotherapy
Pancreatic Cancer		Abdominal pain, often through to the back	Surgery, radiation, chemotherapy
Liver Cancer		Pain in left upper abdomen	Surgery
Colon Cancer	Early	Change in bowel habits, blood in stool	Surgery
	Late	Spread to liver	Chemotherapy

Rectal Cancer	Early	Blood in stool, constipation	Surgery, radiation
	Late	Same	Chemotherapy
Brain Tumors		Headache, visual problems, paralysis— resembles stroke	Surgery, radiation
Ovarian Cancer	Early	Often silent	Surgery, chemotherapy
	Late	Abdominal swelling	
Testicular Cancer		Testicular lump	Surgery + chemotherapy
Lymphoma		Enlarged glands	Chemotherapy, radiation therapy
Hodgkin's Disease		Same	Same
Non-Hodgkin's Disease		Same	Chemotherapy, radiation therapy, bone marrow transplant
Leukemia		Anemia, pallor, fatigue	Chemotherapy, bone marrow transplant
Multiple Myeloma		Diffuse bone pain	Chemotherapy, radiation therapy
Sarcoma		Lumps, swellings	Surgery, chemotherapy, radiation therapy

What to Remember about Cancer

1. The risk of cancer increases with age.
2. The key to the cure of cancer is early detection.
3. Although the cause of cancer is not fully understood, the major role appears to be some abnormality in gene structure.
4. The control of several risk factors for cancer can reduce the incidence of the disease.
5. Tobacco is a major villain in the causation of many cancers.
6. A diet rich in fruits, vegetables, and fiber and low in fat protects against several forms of cancer.
7. The mainstays of cancer treatment continue to be surgery, radiation, and chemotherapy, but newer approaches, such as biological, immunological, and other types, are promising.
8. There are more than 300 new drugs and vaccines currently being tested against all types of cancer.

3

CONSTIPATION

This Chapter Will Really Move You

The scene: A coronary intensive care unit

The time: 11 P.M.

Dr. Schwartz, the cardiology resident, and Miss Tompkins, the charge nurse on duty, enter the coronary care unit. The four patients currently there have all recently suffered heart attacks. The stentorian breathing of the patients breaks the silence of the darkened room. The doctor and nurse study the readings on the monitors as they move from bed to bed, "eyeballing" each patient. They all appear to be sleeping and in no distress; the ECG tracings, blood pressures, and oxygen levels look good. Reassured, they are about to leave the unit when Mr. Smith, in bed number three, calls out, "Doctor, Doctor!" Dr. Schwartz moves quickly to his bedside.

"What is it, sir?" he asked anxiously, knowing that these critically ill patients can be stable one moment and "crash" the next.

"Doctor, I'm in trouble, big trouble."

"No, you're not, Mr. Smith, you're fine. Your ECG is stable and your blood pressure is good. The worst is over," Dr. Schwartz reassures him. "What's worrying you? Are you having chest pain? Are you short of breath?" He looks carefully at the monitor again. Everything is stable.

"No, Doctor, it's nothing like that. But, still I'm very concerned."

"Why, Mr. Smith? What is it? What's wrong?"

"Doctor," Mr. Smith says, his voice choking with emotion, "I didn't move my bowels even once all day today! Yesterday was okay, but today—nothing."

I have witnessed such scenarios scores of times in my many years as a cardiologist. They reflect the fixation on the bowels and their "movement" by every age group, every ethnicity, and every segment of the population, in every part of the country. The enemy is not cramps, diarrhea, or gas, not even Saddam Hussein. It's constipation! "I didn't 'move' today" dominates the psyches of millions of Americans.

I rarely take time out for lunch at my office. I have a salad and a cup of coffee while I talk with my patients. What do you think they discuss as I lift my fork to my mouth or sip my coffee? "You should see my stool, Doctor." They have no hesitation discussing every detail of their bowel habits while I'm eating. "I have these cramps, Doctor, and they move from here to here. I have to strain to get anything out." Obviously I don't relish discussing these details at lunchtime, but since the subject has been raised, it's my job to follow through. So I ask, "What's the color of your movement, Mrs. Brown, once it does come out? And is it narrow like a ribbon?" (A narrow, rib-bonlike stool, associated with constipation, may be a sign of bowel cancer.) Mrs. Brown looks at me with disgust. "Doctor, I wouldn't know. You don't really expect me to look into the toilet bowl, do you?" (If she'd ever taken her dog for a walk, she'd have noticed that it always in-spects what other dogs have left behind. Nature expects it of dogs—and people!)

I don't know how or why this national preoccupation with constipation began. Now that communism is no longer a threat, we seem to need some other "movement" on which to focus, and our bowel conveniently provides it. If we're too busy to think about constipation during the day, we're sure to be reminded of it by friendly television announcers invading the privacy of our bedroom by ped-dling laxatives.

The belief that there are poisons in our stools (the con-stipation mavens call them "toxins") sustains the obses-sion with constipation—"Unless you get rid of them promptly, you're in trouble." My mother, the insomniac (see Chapter 8), was a great authority on these "autotox-ins." As I rushed to leave for school in the morning, she'd wave good-bye to me from the door and invariably shout, "Did you 'sit' this morning?" If I hadn't "sat," she'd pur-sue the matter when I got home in the evening. Her in-terest was not scatological. She was convinced, as are many people, that unless one eliminates every single day, some terrible stuff will be absorbed from the bowel and do you in. Nothing could be farther from the truth. Feces consist of food that hasn't been absorbed. There's no poison in a carload.

Mothers and other laypersons are not the only ones who focus on the stool. Some doctors do, too. There is one specialist in particular, Dr. Anthony Leeds, of King's College in London, who is convinced that the characteristics of your stool are reliable and sophisticated indicators of your health. I'm not talking about obvious changes such as diarrhea, or a severe narrowing of the caliber of the stool, or the presence of mucus or blood. The importance of all these is appreciated by every physician. Dr. Leeds goes much farther. He and his colleagues have constructed a chart displaying the models of different stools—"smooth soft sausages" or "fluffy pieces with ragged edges." He believes that doctors don't ask and patients don't volunteer enough information about their stool characteristics, and as a result the important diagnostic clues are lost. (He should join me for lunch sometime in my office!) To the best of my knowledge, his Bristol Stool Chart (named after the city where it was constructed) is not widely used in this country. But if you're interested in having one in your home, say attached to your refrigerator door, ask your doctor to write to Dr. Leeds for further information.

Concern with constipation, real, perceived, or imagined, is five times more common over the age of sixty-five than in younger adults, even though the aging process itself doesn't really alter bowel function per se. One-third of all healthy, elderly people use laxatives regularly. However, many of those who are convinced that they're constipated usually are not. (When such persons are given laxative placebos, 60 percent of them respond with a bowel movement!) Other laxative users don't really think they're constipated, but they take the medication anyway because they feel the need to have a regular purging.

What Is Constipation?

Officially, you're constipated if you have no more than two bowel movements a week—easily or after straining. But try telling that to Mr. Smith in the coronary care unit, or to any of the millions who are convinced they've got a bowel problem. A more reasonable (and acceptable) definition is "the need to strain at stool, and an ongoing reduction in the number of bowel movements." Remember that the need for daily elimination is not written in stone. Your elimination pattern depends on your diet, how much liquid you consume, your metabolism level, the medications you're taking, the elimination habits you formed early in life, and whether or not you have any underlying medical problems. Many healthy people move their bowels every day; others do so every second day; some have only one motion a day; others have two or three. But a sudden reduction in the frequency of pattern may, indeed, reflect constipation. If this state of affairs continues for a week or two and there is no obvious explanation, tell your doctor about it. Sudden cessation of bowel movements accompanied by nausea, vomiting, severe belly pain, or a feeling of fullness soon after eating may be due to intestinal obstruction, and that's a real emergency. Call your doctor immediately!

Constipation without Mechanical Blockage

The food we eat passes through the stomach, which removes and absorbs many of the essential nutrients. What's left then enters the small intestine, where further absorption occurs. The residue ends up as stool (feces) in the large bowel (colon)—the last four to six feet of the gut. The colon normally absorbs most of the two quarts of water along with minerals and other nutrients that it receives each day from the small intestine. This reabsorption of water by the bowel is critical. Unless it occurs, the water is excreted and we become dehydrated. Feces, which are nothing more than waste products from what we've eaten that we either don't need or can't absorb, are propelled down the bowel by the contraction of muscles in its wall. This muscular activity is automatic, that is, it's effected by stimulation of the involuntary or autonomic nervous system—the same nerves that regulate our heartbeat, breathing, perspiration, and so on. Happily, bowel contraction does not require any deliberate action on our part. If it did, we'd have to sit there all day concentrating on moving things along. When bowel function goes awry, as it sometimes does in nerve disorders in diabetics and in certain stroke patients, constipation results.

When the feces have filled the sigmoid (the left side of the lower colon) and there is no room for more, they move down into the rectum, ready to be excreted. That's when you get the signal to head for the bathroom. Fortunately, the muscles at the anus are under your voluntary control, so that if you're held up in traffic or in the middle of some important business and can't answer the call to eliminate immediately, the anal sphincter will hold the fort until you can.

But if the bowel reabsorbs too much water, or you take a diuretic (which makes you pass large amounts of urine), or you're dehydrated because you haven't been drinking enough liquids, the stool becomes hard and dry. *Voilà*— constipation.

Risk Factors for Constipation

The most common causes of constipation at any age are too little fiber and not enough liquids in the diet. However, as you get older, other contributing factors come into play. These include the following:

• **Lack of exercise:** This is happening much less often as older people begin to appreciate the importance of keeping fit. Regular exercise prevents constipation by increasing the contractions of the intestine.

• **Medication:** People tend to take more drugs as they get older, and many of them are constipating. Among the common offenders are iron supplements (they make the stool hard and black), calcium supplements, diuretics (water pills), and antidepressants (especially the tricyclics, of which Elavil is the prototype) and other mood-altering drugs that reduce the contractility of the muscle in the bowel wall. Other culprits are chemotherapy agents such as vincristine and vinblastine that interfere with function of the autonomic nervous system (see above); painkillers (particularly those with narcotics such as codeine that slow the bowel down); antacids, especially Pepto-Bismol and those that contain aluminum (check their labels for these ingredients); nonsteroidal anti-inflammatory drugs (the prototype of which is ibuprofen), which block prostaglandin and so inhibit bowel contractions; calcium channel blockers, notably verapamil, nifedipine, and diltiazem (all of which reduce the motility of smooth muscle in the bowel); ACE inhibitors used in the treatment of high blood pressure (the prototype is captopril [Capoten]) that inhibit the relaxation of bowel muscle; and many others. If your bowel habits change after you start taking any new medication, especially those listed above, consult your doctor.

• **Depression** can be a serious problem in the elderly (see Chapter 4), and constipation is one of its consequences. Someone who's depressed may ignore the urge to empty the bowels, or the antidepressants they're taking may slow bowel activity. Decreased food intake for any reason, like loss of appetite or the side effect of certain medications such as digitalis, can also lead to constipation.

• **Diabetes** takes a toll in two major areas of the body, the blood vessels and the nerves, especially if sugar levels have been poorly controlled. The vascular consequences are hardening of the arteries; the complication of nerve involvement is called "autonomic dysfunction," in which the involuntary nerve function that controls bowel motility becomes impaired. (The stimuli that cause the muscles to contract and propel waste products down and out don't work properly.) The result is a sluggish bowel—and constipation. Diabetes can also cause constipation, but in another way. When the blood sugar level is high, the kidneys try to help out by eliminating excess sugar in the urine. But since they can't pass sugar cubes, they need water in which to dissolve the sugar. This absorption leaves less water for the stool, which then becomes dry and harder to eliminate.

• **Hypothyroidism** (an underactive thyroid gland) causes a slowing down of all our body functions because the thyroid gland controls metabolism. Constipation is a prominent symptom of hypothyroidism. This diagnosis is very often missed, especially when the symptoms are subtle. I don't know how many millions of people go through life tired, overweight, sluggish—and constipated—because they lack thyroid hormone, which can be so easily replaced.

• **Diverticulosis and diverticulitis** are both the result and cause of constipation. Diverticula are fingerlike projections from the wall of the bowel. They are especially common in people and cultures where constipation is prevalent and fiber is low in the diet. Straining at a hard stool leads to increased pressure within the bowel, causing portions of its wall to extrude and form pockets (diverticula). As long as these pockets are not infected, the condition is called diverticulosis. However, when they become inflamed or infected, the disorder is called diverticulitis, and is characterized by pain, low-grade fever, and, again, constipation. We used to think that this inflammation occurred when seeds or other tiny food particles became imbedded in the diverticula and irritated them. So for years, doctors advised these patients to eat soft diets and avoid seeds. This was wrong, and we currently prescribe the opposite kind of diet—one rich in fiber, in order to prevent constipation, which is the underlying cause of this condition.

• **Stroke** and other neurological abnormalities such as Parkinson's disease that specifically affect the elderly, as well as spinal cord injuries and multiple sclerosis, which usually occur in younger people, can cause either constipation or incontinence. Constipation results when the "time to go" signal is either misinterpreted or never sent because of brain damage. Incontinence, the inability to control the bowels, occurs when the anal sphincter nerves that keep the feces from exiting don't function properly.

Older people with a neurological problem that's left them weak or paralyzed often don't move around very much. When you're sedentary, your bowels are less likely to move normally. That's why we give stool softeners to patients in hospital who are confined to bed rest for whatever reason.

• **Chronic laxative abuse:** The same people who feel the need to purge themselves with enemas (come hell or high water) or laxatives ultimately develop a bowel that will only function when pushed to do so. As time goes on, the need for such stimulation increases, as does their constipation.

• **Generalized weakness** leaves the abdominal muscles unable to force the stool out effectively. This is especially true in older people. The abdominal muscles are also less strong in patients with severe emphysema.

• **Frequent travel and on-the-run eating habits** that make it difficult to heed nature's call frequently cause chronic constipation, increased pressure in the colon, and diverticulosis.

Although constipation is usually the result of correctable lifestyle aspects, more ominous reasons account for the 100,000 admissions to hospital each year for constipation-based problems. A tumor of the bowel causing mechanical obstruction is the greatest worry in someone with sudden onset of constipation. Not every tumor is malignant; many are benign polyps, which, if large enough, can also cause obstruction.

You should suspect a bowel tumor whenever you observe a change in caliber of the stool, which becomes narrower after passing through the obstructed area; the presence of blood in the stool, not always visible to the naked eye (that's why the doctor will perform chemical tests to detect it in your stool specimen); and a hard, infrequent stool often alternating with diarrhea. Bloating, abdominal pain, intermittent cramping, and the feeling of incomplete emptying of your colon after a movement are other signs suggestive of trouble.

Tumors are not the only causes of obstruction. Scar tissue (adhesions) after abdominal surgery or radiation to the belly can form around the colon and interfere with its normal function. This tissue may need to be freed up by surgery.

• **Irritable Bowel Syndrome (IBS)** usually begins earlier in life, but it can also affect the elderly. People with IBS have a variety of intestinal complaints, the most common of which are cramps, diarrhea, gas, and bloating. However, they may also suffer from constipation. The frustrating thing about IBS is that all the tests done to evaluate these symptoms usually come back normal, so these poor folks get very little sympathy for their misery. Treatment isn't very satisfactory, either. The reassurance that the constellation of intestinal symptoms is not inflammatory bowel disease (IBD, see below) is the most comforting thing a doctor can tell someone with IBS. Treatment consists of following a high-fiber diet, especially when constipation is the main complaint; avoidance of milk and milk products (since many of these patients are lactose deficient); and symptomatic treatment of the symptoms. Unfortunately, there is no cure for this affliction. Although this disorder won't shorten your life, it can make you miserable.

• **Inflammatory Bowel Disease (IBD)** refers either to ulcerative colitis or regional enteritis (Crohn's disease). Don't confuse it with IBS, which is described above. Although these two disorders have many symptoms in common, including intermittent constipation, IBD can be life-threatening, while IBS virtually never is. The colon is chronically inflamed in IBD, probably due to some malfunction of the autoimmune system. Like IBS, this disorder affects primarily the young, but it can also develop later in life.

Preventing Constipation

The first rule to prevent constipation is to heed nature's signals. If you ignore them often enough, the messages stop coming, and you will end up constipated. Give yourself plenty of time to move your bowels; don't rush or become impatient. If you're older and your abdominal muscles are weak so that you have trouble expelling a hard stool, you can make them work more effectively by elevating your legs while you're on the toilet.

• **Drink lots of fluids** (at least eight glasses a day, and ten in hot weather). To help you get the amount of water you need, drink a whole glass, not just a sip, whenever you take a pill. Plain water is preferable to other liquids such as juices, sodas, coffee, tea, or beer, especially if you're diabetic, because it contains no calories. A glass of water with the juice of half a lemon, or four to six ounces of prune juice in the morning, will help your bowel get going.

• **Adequate fiber intake** is as important as enough water in preventing constipation. It increases the transit time within the bowel so that the waste products get down and out more quickly. The richest sources of fiber are unprocessed grains, such as bran, which is usually eaten in bread and cereals. However, the problem with bran is that it leaves you gassier than some of the other grains. But beans, fresh fruits, and vegetables (asparagus, brussels sprouts, cabbage, and carrots are especially good), and dried fruits, such as raisins, prunes, and apricots, are all effective too.

Most people know how important fiber is, not only for the control of constipation, but also to prevent cancer. Yet for some reason, Americans still eat only a fraction of the thirty-five or forty grams of fiber we need every day.

Once you've decided to go the fiber route, you may have some side effects during the first two or three weeks—bloating, flatulence, and irregular bowel movements. But stick with it. You'll be glad you did when your bowels start moving normally and regularly. Remember, fiber is filling and low in calories, so it also helps control your weight; soluble fiber (found primarily in oat cereal, oat bran, barley, and a variety of legumes) also lowers cholesterol.

Treating Constipation

If your constipation is the result of a growth, either a benign polyp or a cancer, none of the following measures will do much good. The treatment for physical obstruction is its removal. However, functional disturbances of the bowel do respond to medication.

THE SCOOP ON LAXATIVES

Laxatives are big business, with a market of about $400 million a year in this country. However, they're better for the manufacturer than they are for you. Avoid them for as long as you can. Their long-term use can weaken your abdominal muscles which are no longer called upon to do even the normal amount of work to expel the stool; they leave the colon lazy, and they can cause the loss of vitamins, minerals, and other vital nutrients. Before resorting to laxatives, increase your fiber intake, drink more water, and start a regular exercise program. If you do need "help," take the mildest preparation, for the shortest length of time.

There are several different categories of laxatives; some of which are safer and more effective than others. The most widely used in this country are the following:

Bulk laxatives, both natural and synthetic, account for 25 percent of all laxative sales. They are essentially some form of fiber, and they work by drawing water into the bowel. This makes the stool larger, softer, and easier to expel. The best known of these substances is Metamucil, an indigestible fiber (hemicellulose) derived from the seeds of the psyllium plant. Others are Citrucel and Serutan (in case you haven't noticed, Serutan is "Natures" spelled backwards). These bulk laxatives can cause impaction (hardening) of the stool and obstruct your bowel, so be sure to take each dose with a full glass of water. Bulk laxatives are safer over the long term than are the stimulant laxatives. In addition, they have the added benefit of decreasing the formation of diverticula. The main drawback to their long-term use is their interference with the absorption of other medications you require. So don't take any other drugs at the same time as a bulk laxative. Wait an hour or two.

Dried kidney beans are an excellent fiber laxative. A half-cup of cooked beans costs less than a dime, contains eight grams of fat, and is not only a laxative, but is also rich in vitamins, proteins, minerals, and carbohydrates.

Saline laxatives draw fluid into your large bowel, increase the pressure within it, and leave your stool wetter, softer, and easier to eliminate. The usual salts saline laxatives contain are phosphates, citrates, sulfates, and magnesium, and the best-known name brand is probably Milk of Magnesia. Saline laxatives usually work within three hours, which is why they're preferred for cleaning out the colon before surgery, sigmoidoscopy, colonoscopy, or after a bowel X ray to get rid of the barium. They should only be used for such one-time situations, and never on an ongoing basis. Avoid them as you would any salt if you have high blood pressure, kidney problems, or heart failure.

Stimulant laxatives account for 25 percent of all "bowel regulators" sold in this country, and they should be your last resort. They work by irritating the lining of the colon so that it contracts and expels its contents. They can produce unpleasant side effects, such as cramping soon after they're taken, especially in older people. When used regularly, they can result in dependence, vitamin deficiency, and loss of nutrients. The most widely used of these laxatives is castor oil (shades of my childhood), which I do not recommend because it can interfere with the absorption of dietary nutrients. Others are bisacodyl, of which the best-known brand names are Dulcolax, senna (Senokot), Correctol, Purge, Feen-A-Mint, and the old standby, Ex-Lax. Most of these are available as tablets or suppositories. The tablets have a protective coating, which prevents their absorption in the stomach. Don't chew or crush them, because they can damage the tissues of your mouth and stomach. Antacids, milk, cimetidine (Tagamet), or any drug that prevents acid formation dissolve the protective enteric coating of these stimulant laxatives, so take them at least an hour apart. Don't be alarmed if the senna laxative turns your urine brown or violet. This color change is harmless. Phenolphthalein used to be a main constituent of Ex-Lax and other brands, but is now banned by the FDA because it was shown to cause cancer in rodents in very high doses.

Enemas are a way of life for many people. I have no objection to an occasional enema to correct an acute problem. However, high colonics at regular intervals, in my view, are a fad. Its devotees insist I'm wrong. They say they feel so "clean" after one of these treatments. I think it's only a state of mind. Don't let anyone tell you that it removes "toxins." None have even been found. Enemas remove stool, yes; toxins, no. Your bowel has the wherewithal to cleanse itself. The bowel sheds its lining every twenty-four hours without the need for the ritual high colonic. Sending in ten or fifteen gallons of water only upsets its normal function.

Stool softeners are not laxatives. They won't move you, but your stool will be softer when you do go. We give stool softeners to people who are going to be laid up for a while after an injury, operation, or for any other reason. Many patients continue taking them after they leave the hospital. Unlike laxatives, there is no danger in doing so indefinitely; just make sure they don't leave your stool so soft that it slips out when you least expect it. The prototype of these softeners is sodium docusate, marketed as Colace. Other brand names are Surfak and Dialose.

Many older people use mineral oil to lubricate their bowel and to keep their stools soft. I prefer Colace. Mineral oil is a softener *and* a laxative and does make it easier for you to pass your stool. However, the oil prevents the absorption of the important fat-soluble vitamins (A, D, E, and K) and may leave you deficient in them. An older person who is weak and bed-bound, and whose swallowing mechanism is not quite as strong as it should be, can inadvertently inhale the mineral oil in the lung while trying to swallow it, and end up with "lipoid" (fat) pneumonia. This condition is hard to treat because the culprit is fat in the lung and not a bacteria or virus that can be cured by an antibiotic. And mineral oil also has a habit of leaking out of your anus, soiling your clothes. So all in all, I suggest you stay away from mineral oil. However, if you're determined to use it, here are some important precautions: Take it rectally rather than by the oral route. If you do take it by mouth, do so at bedtime on an empty stomach, and never with a stool softener such as Colace. The latter causes increased absorption of the mineral oil into your body.

How Doctors Evaluate Constipation

To evaluate your constipation, the first and most obvious step is a good history. The details of when and why your problem started, and whether there are any aspects of your lifestyle or medical history that can explain it, are very important. Your doctor will also examine the stool, looking mainly for evidence of blood. A careful physical exam that includes blood tests, which may provide other clues, is vital. This exam must include a digital rectal examination. I was taught long ago in medical school that if "you don't put your finger in, you put your foot in." A rectal allows the doctor to determine the tone of the muscle that opens and shuts the anus (anal sphincter), and it can reveal any areas of tenderness, tumors low down in the intestinal tract, hemorrhoids, or blood.

If these noninvasive steps do not determine the cause of your constipation, a "look-see" into the bowel is usually the next step. Modern instruments for this purpose are so thin and flexible that the procedures can be done with little or no discomfort. You'll also, of course, receive some sedation. The older scopes were large and rigid, so patients and doctors used to prefer to do a barium enema first. But that was messy, involved exposure to radiation, provided only an indirect picture of what was going on, and didn't permit the biopsy of any growths that were found. So these days you're apt to have a colonoscopy, which allows the doctor to view the entire colon. Some doctors do a sigmoidoscopy instead, in which they introduce the scope into the lower portion of the bowel, rather than throughout its entire length.

The night before the test, you'll drink a saline laxative (described above). My own gastroenterologist uses a preparation called Golytely. (If you've ever taken it, you know what a misnomer it is!) These laxatives clean the bowel so the doctor can get a clear view of its interior and thus detect any polyps or other growths.

The thin and flexible colonoscope has a light at its end, and forceps with which to snare or snip any suspicious tissue that is seen. This instrument is longer than that employed for sigmoidoscopy because it goes the entire length of the bowel.

Complications of Chronic Constipation

Straining at stools is not only a nuisance and an inconvenience, it can also be a big pain in the you-know-what. It can also lead to hemorrhoids (painful swelling of the veins in the anal and rectal area, sometimes resulting in chronic bleeding or oozing from the area); the skin around the anus can become stretched and tear, causing painful fissures; chronic forcing to eliminate stool can permit a small portion of the intestinal lining to be extruded from the anal opening, a condition called rectal prolapse. It's also often accompanied by mucus leaking from the bowel.

When constipation is so severe and the stool so hard that you simply can't push it out, you've got fecal impaction. The feces then usually require softening with a lubricant such as mineral oil, and the doctor or nurse then needs to break them up with the finger and remove them. Fecal impaction, especially in an older person, is more than just an advanced case of constipation. It is an emergency, which, if untreated, can lead to cardiac, circulatory, and respiratory symptoms—and even death.

What to Remember about Constipation

1. You probably don't have constipation, even if you think you do.
2. Constipation is defined as two or less bowel movements a week. However, any continuing decrease in the number of your movements, especially accompanied by a hard, dry stool, is indicative of constipation.
3. Most cases of constipation are due to one's lifestyle, not disease. The most important contributing factors are too little water and fiber in the diet.
4. Laxatives should be used only briefly, and as a last resort while you retrain yourself and your bowel. The safest among them are the bulk laxatives that contain fiber.

5. There are certain predisposing conditions for constipation, such as weak abdominal walls, stroke, diverticulitis, medications, diabetes, and others, described above.

6. Persistent constipation, especially when alternating with diarrhea or accompanied by a change in the stool size or shape, should be investigated.

4

DEPRESSION

When Clouds Have Lost
Their Silver Lining

There is an epidemic of depression in this country. Almost 30 million Americans, more than 10 percent of the population, are chronically depressed or suffer from some related mood disorder. This includes an unspecified number of menopausal women and about 6 million persons over the age of sixty-five. These numbers are probably a low estimate because so many of us aren't really aware that we're depressed, or we're ashamed to admit it, or we believe we're too old to be helped. That's all the more tragic since depression can be improved by treatment in 70 to 90 percent of cases, at any age, regardless of the cause.

Depressed patients spend 50 percent more money on medical bills than the average person; they visit their doctor or go to the emergency room more often, they undergo more tests, receive more prescriptions, and remain in hospitals longer than is usually necessary. Study after study has shown that depression slows recovery from any illness, aggravates its symptoms, and hastens death. You might think that many of these stricken people welcome escape from their suffering. But that's apparently not so. In a recent large study, the majority of persons in their eighties who were asked whether they would prefer a shorter life of better quality or a longer one in chronic pain opted for a longer life. They were prepared to suffer so long as they could continue to be with their loved ones. However, between 1980 and 1982, the incidence of suicide among persons age sixty-five and older increased by 9 percent; and in those eighty to eighty-four, it rose by a staggering 35 percent! Even more frightening is the fact that most people who kill themselves visit their doctor in the month before doing so, and fully 40 percent commit suicide within seven days of that visit! Doctors apparently do not recognize most cases of depression severe enough to lead to suicide.

I am not a psychiatrist, and this is not a chapter on psychiatric problems of the aging population. However, I can tell you this: Depression—the continued, overwhelming feelings of sadness and despair that interfere with normal living—is not an inevitable accompaniment to growing old. There's nothing about the biochemistry or biology of aging that causes it.

Many older people have good reason to be depressed. They may have lost a spouse or some close friends and relatives and suddenly become aware of their own mortality (the "it's only a matter of time" frame of mind). They dwell on the fact that their number will soon be up, and they wonder how it will all end. Something every day reminds them that they're here on earth only as tenants, not landlords. Making a will never used to bother me. I remember how nonchalantly I signed one shortly after my first child was born some forty years ago. Preparing for the end of my life then was so theoretical. But now . . .

There are many reasons to be sad and depressed other than the expectation of death. If you're pushing sixty-five or have passed it, you probably know what I mean. Maybe you were told that you must retire, even though you feel great, want to work, and can use the money. No one else will hire you; you're too old. So you now face the transition from an active, productive life to that of a retired senior citizen. If you have a good-sized nest egg and hobbies, you'll adjust after a while. But older people without a steady income often cannot maintain the standard of living to which they had become accustomed and have even taken for granted. The shock is buffered to some extent if they're living at home, with a spouse or other family. But there are millions of older people who have no one to turn to, who are confined to hospitals or nursing homes because of frailty, dementia, or chronic disease. At least half of them are seriously depressed. Can you blame them?

What helps tip the scale toward depression in any one of these scenarios is the onset of some disease that's painful and/or life-threatening, or that robs older people of their independence: They can't hear well; they can't see clearly; they can't remember; they've had a heart attack; their joints are stiff; sex is only a memory; they either can't pee and have to be rushed to an emergency room every now and then to have their urine removed by a catheter, or they have to "go" every few minutes. Or perhaps a previously active, self-sufficient man or woman may be left paralyzed after a stroke and can no longer speak or get around without help. Are any of these people apt to be depressed? You'd better believe it.

But there's a difference between appropriate sadness in response to misfortune and depression that needs to be treated. Most people, at any age, adjust and continue to function in the face of adversity. Of course they're sad from time to time. That's normal. But they "bounce back" and carry on. The ability to do so is very important. This chapter discusses how to recognize true depression, and the best way to deal with it.

Symptoms of Depression

There is a spectrum of depression. At the one end there is the self-limiting sadness provoked by some personal tragedy; at the other there is the melancholy that persists, often without an apparent cause. Regrettably, doctors and family members don't always understand the difference between the two extremes.

Whether a depression needs treatment depends on how severe and disabling it is. There are no hard and fixed definitions for these designations. If you're depressed for an obvious reason and your symptoms persist for weeks or longer, a mild antidepressant will often help. If you remain depressed for more than two months or your depression comes and goes, you may require treatment indefinitely.

Older people usually manifest their depression by being withdrawn and listless, with no interest in anything or anyone. (Younger persons are more apt to be agitated, restless, or anxious.) Here are some of the symptoms to look for in the elderly:

- **Ongoing sadness or anxiety.**
- **Trouble concentrating or making decisions,** such as what to wear or what to buy. Thoughts drift while reading, conversing, or watching TV. When asked a question, they may not answer, or they respond with "Don't bother me" or "I don't know."
- **Loss of interest in activities** that were formerly important and gave pleasure; neglect of hobbies and homes.
- **No interest in sex** after a lifelong strong libido.
- **Irritability or a change in personality;** a previously fastidious person neglects his or her appearance, for example.
- **Excessive crying,** often for no apparent reason.
- **Change in sleep patterns**—either insomnia or excessive drowsiness.
- **Feelings of hopelessness, worthlessness, or guilt.** Some event in the distant past, long forgotten by everyone else involved, is recollected as a bad deed deserving punishment. Some of these feelings of expiation may stem from the expectation of impending death, and possible punishment in the hereafter for a transgression, real or imagined, earlier in life.

- **Inability to function** at work or at home.
- **Someone who is depressed, doesn't hear well, and has poor vision** may become paranoid, feel persecuted, and believe that there is a conspiracy against him.
- **Chronic fatigue** or lack of energy.
- **Unexplained aches and pains,** especially headaches, constipation, and weight loss.
- **Change in appetite,** either a loss of hunger or compulsive eating.
- **Thoughts of death or suicide.**
- **Memory loss.** Although many middle-aged adults will occasionally forget names or words and say "Now, why did I come into this room?" these memory lapses are more frequent in older people and cause more intense reactions.

The signs of depression are not always classical, like those listed above. Sometimes you have to be attuned to them. My father's brother is a case in point. Uncle David was my favorite uncle, and I his favorite nephew; he had no children of his own. He was a brilliant actor, a great mimic, and one of the funniest people I had ever met. When he was in his mid-seventies, those of us who knew him best began to note a subtle change in his behavior. It was nothing you could point to and say "Uncle David is depressed." He seemed a little less spontaneous and not quite as argumentative (he used to enjoy playing the devil's advocate). One evening I realized how depressed he really was. He had invited me for dinner—just the two of us. After some small talk, he became very serious. "Here, I want you to have this," he said, and gave me his gold wristwatch. I had never seen Uncle David without this watch. He'd had it as long as I could remember, and I knew what it meant to him. It had been given to him when he left an acting company in Moscow where he lived before emigrating to Palestine. "But why give this to me? Did you get another watch from someone?" "No," he said, "how much longer will I need it? You'll have more use for it than I will." Older people divesting themselves prematurely of their treasured possessions is often a sign of depression, signaling a hopelessness and a belief that there is no future.

The Geriatric Depression Scale (Short Form)

If you wonder whether you're depressed, or suspect it in an elderly friend or relative, check it out on this Geriatric Depression Scale.

Choose the best answer for how you felt over the past week:

1. Are you basically satisfied with your life?   Yes/No

2. Have you dropped many of your activities
   and interests?   Yes/No

3. Do you feel that your life is empty?   Yes/No

4. Do you often get bored?   Yes/No

5. Are you in good spirits most of the time? Yes/No

6. Are you afraid that something bad is going to happen to you? Yes/No

7. Do you feel happy most of the time? Yes/No

8. Do you often feel helpless? Yes/No

9. Do you prefer to stay at home, rather than going out and doing new things? Yes/No

10. Do you feel that you have more problems with memory than most? Yes/No

11. Do you think it is wonderful to be alive now? Yes/No

12. Do you feel pretty worthless the way you are now? Yes/No

13. Do you feel full of energy? Yes/No

14. Do you feel that your situation is hopeless? Yes/No

15. Do you think that most people are better off than you are? Yes/No

Each of the following answers counts as one point. A score greater than five indicates probable depression.

1. No	6. Yes	11. No
2. Yes	7. No	12. Yes
3. Yes	8. Yes	13. No
4. Yes	9. Yes	14. Yes
5. No	10. Yes	15. Yes

Make Sure It's Depression

The most typical case of depression may sometimes reflect and accompany some other disease. Forty to fifty percent of people diagnosed with an emotional or psychiatric disorder, including depression, turn out to have an undiagnosed physical ailment. Never assume that any set of symptoms necessarily means depression in an older person. You may end up neglecting a treatable condition. Anyone who is depressed, with or without an obvious reason, deserves a thorough medical evaluation as well as a mental status exam by a qualified specialist. The following are examples of disorders that can be mistaken for depression:

• **About 40 percent of patients with Parkinson's disease** also have serious depression. When they don't have the telltale tremor, the other stigmata of their disease—the fixed expression, stooped posture, slow movements, and a quiet, monotonous voice—may be mistaken for depression. Of course, many patients with Parkinson's disease are also depressed, in which case they require therapy for both conditions.

• **We tend to think of stroke** mainly in terms of residual paralysis, yet more than 30 percent of stroke victims are depressed. This is most likely to happen when the left side of the brain has been damaged in right-handed people, causing weakness or paralysis of the right side of the body—and vice versa in left-handed people with right-sided brain damage.

• **As you would expect, 40 percent of patients with cancer** are depressed. I'm surprised the figure isn't much higher. Many cancer patients are better able to cope with their disease when given antidepressants along with whatever other drugs they need.

• **The lowered metabolism in hypothyroidism** causes symptoms that can be mistaken for evidence of depression: mental and physical slowing, poor memory, an apathetic demeanor, fatigue, and constipation. All it takes to make the right diagnosis is a high index of suspicion and a simple blood test.

• **Polymyalgia rheumatica and temporal arteritis,** related diseases of the autoimmune system, are common in older people and are associated with profound fatigue, headache, and unexplained loss of appetite, all of which suggest depression. Treatment with steroids cures both these disorders. (Temporal arteritis can lead to blindness or stroke if left untreated.)

• **Half the patients with Alzheimer's disease** are also depressed. I suspect it if they suddenly stop eating and their other symptoms worsen. In such cases, an antidepressant may reverse what was thought to be an inexorable progression of their Alzheimer's.

• **Various drugs** can interact poorly and cause depression, so be sure to review every medication whenever that diagnosis is suspected, regardless of whether it was prescribed by your doctor or you bought it yourself over-the-counter or at a health-food store. This is especially true in older people who may be taking several medications.

- **Anemia** makes you tired, and when you have less energy you may appear to be depressed.
- **Increased alcohol intake** or withdrawal can leave you somnolent or combative, with mood swings easily mistaken for depression.

The following commonly used medications can cause depression:

- **Antihypertensive agents** (to lower elevated blood pressure). Among the most widely prescribed are the beta-blockers such as propranolol, atenolol, and metoprolol. I first noted this effect some twenty-five years ago, and reported it at the time to the head of the National Heart Institute. Beta-blockers should not be the first choice for treating hypertension, especially in persons over sixty. I always start with a diuretic (water pill).

- **Steroids** are widely prescribed for a variety of diseases, including severe asthma, arthritis, cancer, autoimmune disorders, and for the prevention of organ rejection. Anyone taking a daily dose of 20 milligrams or more of prednisone (the prototype of steroids) has a one-in-three chance of developing behavioral problems, including depression. If you need steroids, take the lowest effective dose for no longer than is absolutely necessary.

- **Drugs for Parkinson's disease,** especially the most widely used ones in the levodopa family, often cause depression. Levodopa is the best drug for the treatment of Parkinson's. Unfortunately, even if it results in depression it must be continued because there is no effective alternative therapy. In that case, take antidepressant drugs along with it. This is a rare example of having to accommodate to an agent with known side effects because there is no other treatment available.

• **Painkillers and sleeping pills,** alone or in combination, are notorious causes of depression in the elderly. So are some of the over-the-counter antihistamines that promise you a good night's sleep (unless they shut down your bladder so that you can't pee if you have a large prostate). Your first line of drugs for pain relief should be aspirin, acetaminophen (Tylenol), and the nonsteroidal anti-inflammatory drugs (NSAIDs), such as ibuprofen. (See Chapter 8 for the best way to deal with insomnia.)

Treating Depression

When depression persists despite love, reassurance, and support, and treatment is necessary, there are many effective antidepressants from which to choose. Several studies have shown that the combination of drugs and psychotherapy is more effective than either alone. Many older patients do not have either the money or the inclination for ongoing psychiatric care, and few health plans reimburse for it.

Before resorting to the prescription antidepressant agents, I first suggest *Saint-John's-wort* (Hypericum perforatum.) This is a natural substance with no significant side effects (although if you're a sun worshiper—shame—and frequently bask in the harmful ultraviolet rays, you may develop a skin rash if you're on Saint-John's-wort). It is widely used throughout Europe as a mild antidepressant, and its effectiveness is currently being evaluated by the National Institutes of Health. The usual dosage is 900 milligrams a day, and it takes about four weeks to work.

If depression continues unabated despite reassurance, the control of symptoms due to other underlying diseases, and a trial of Saint-John's-wort, I then prescribe a more potent antidepressant. Before doing so, however, I perform a thorough physical examination, paying special attention to how well the patient's kidneys and liver are working. Many of these antidepressant drugs are excreted or handled by these organs, which, if already impaired, can be further damaged by the antidepressant. They can allow toxic levels of these drugs to accumulate in the body. Make sure that your doctor knows about every single medication you're taking before starting *any* antidepressant—these agents can interact with one another, either reducing their effectiveness or causing toxicity. Even the relatively benign Saint-John's-wort should not be used with another antidepressant.

When prescribing any antidepressant, especially to persons over sixty-five, I start with the mildest agent first and give only one-third to one-half the usual dose for the first two to three weeks. I then gradually increase it until I observe the desired effect.

There are several categories of *antidepressants*. The older ones, though still useful in some cases, are not as well tolerated in seniors as are the newer *selective serotonin reuptake inhibitors (SSRIs)*, the best known of which are Prozac, Paxil, and Zoloft (fluoxetine, paroxetine, and sertraline, respectively). These should be the first-line prescription antidepressants for older people.

The SSRIs work by prolonging the activity of serotonin, a chemical in the brain that affects mood and which is often decreased in depressed persons. Their most common side effects are gastrointestinal nausea, diarrhea, and appetite loss. But I have also seen SSRIs cause nervousness, anxiety, tremor, dizziness, insomnia, impaired sexual function, dry mouth, headache, drowsiness, weight loss, flu-like symptoms, and fatigue. Don't let this list scare you off. These complications do not occur frequently and they clear up when you stop the drug.

Though perhaps best known, Prozac is not my first choice because it has a long half-life—that is, it takes several days to be excreted from the body. So if it does cause any troublesome side effects, you'll have to whistle Dixie until it's out of your system. The usual starting dose of Prozac for an older depressed person is 5 to 10 milligrams a day, and it's best to stay with that dose for at least a week before increasing it.

I prefer Paxil and Zoloft to Prozac because they have a half-life of only a day or so. But don't drive if you're taking Paxil, because it can make you drowsy. Zoloft is my favorite antidepressant. One word of caution, however: Zoloft can interfere with warfarin (Coumadin), the anticoagulant. That doesn't mean you can't take the two together; you'll just need to have your blood tested more frequently to make sure that it's neither too thick nor too thin. All the SSRIs can also reduce your sex drive and prevent an orgasm.

If you're given an SSRI, be sure to tell your doctor if you're also taking any medication to lower your blood pressure, or lithium (for manic depression), or dextromethorphan, a common ingredient in over-the-counter cough medicines. For some reason, these drugs interact unfavorably with the SSRIs.

The SSRIs are not necessarily more effective than some of the other older agents, but they're better tolerated and safer. They also have less of a sedative effect. However, if they don't work, of if they produce unacceptable side effects, you do have other options. My first choices among them are nefazodone (Serzone) and venlafaxine (Effexor), both of which act very much like the SSRIs. I don't think they're quite as effective, but they have very few side effects (the most frequent ones being nausea, headache, sleepiness, insomnia, and constipation), and their half-life is only ten hours, so the body eliminates them quickly.

The tricyclics (TCAs), a family of antidepressants that has been around for more than thirty years, continue to be a useful third option. Unfortunately, these otherwise effective agents can cause significant side effects in about 10 percent of patients. They can drop the blood pressure in some patients, leaving them dizzy and vulnerable to falling. (All you need with your depression is a broken hip.) They also occasionally produce cardiac rhythm disturbances and, rarely, even sudden cardiac death. So if you have any heart problems, and especially if you're recovering from a heart attack, avoid this group of drugs. I always do an electrocardiogram on any patient before starting a tricyclic agent. This group of drugs is now being used more and more for control of chronic pain, and less against depression. My preference among them is nortriptyline (Aventyl, Pamelor) because it carries the smallest risk of cardiac complications. The usual dose is anywhere between 10 and 50 milligrams, best taken at night. Its most common side effects are dry mouth, constipation, fatigue, and tremors.

Buproprion, marketed under two names, Wellbutrin and Zyban, is another second-line drug against depression. Zyban is the weaker formulation and is touted as an aid to smoking cessation. If your doctor has prescribed Zyban to help you break the habit but your insurance carrier won't pay for smoking cessation aids, get Wellbutrin and adjust the dosage. (Just another commentary on the strange economics of modern medical practice.) Buproprion for depression is safe in the recommended dose of 300 milligrams a day taken in divided doses. Its most common side effects are agitation, weight loss, dizziness, and a decreased appetite. Higher doses can cause seizures. And by the way, some of my patients have told me that, unlike the SSRIs, buproprion stimulates their sexual appetite.

Compliance with any antidepressant is a major problem. The people for whom they're prescribed are often so depressed they don't take them. That can be dealt with in a hospital or a nursing home, where medication is given to the patient on schedule. However, at home someone must make sure that the prescribed drugs are taken in the right dosage and at the right time. The doctor can help in such cases by prescribing medications such as the SSRIs that need be given only once daily—and that interact least with any other drugs the patient is taking.

Electroconvulsive (electroshock) therapy (ECT) was used widely before the modern antidepressant drugs became available. However, it's still the fastest-acting, most efficient option in cases of depression or severe agitation that have not responded to drug therapy. ECT is often required when something must be done quickly, as, for example, when a depressed patient is starving, agitated, or obviously suicidal. ECT is also useful when patients cannot tolerate the side effects of medications.

A course of ECT usually requires six to twelve treatments, generally two to three times a week at first, then at weekly or longer intervals. And it doesn't hurt. ECT is successful in about 80 to 90 percent of cases, and has no long-term downside. In fact, I think that over the long run, it's safer than most of the tricyclics. It can, however, temporarily impair short-term memory. You can receive the therapy on an outpatient basis, or your doctor may prefer to administer it in the hospital. Here's how it's done: You are asked not to eat or drink anything after midnight. After you receive an anesthetic, the brain is stimulated by an electric current that alters the brain's chemical and electrical activity. These changes improve mood and relieve agitation. The procedure takes about thirty minutes, and you can usually go home the same day. Antidepressants may be prescribed after ECT, but psychiatrists now usually recommend continuation of ECT once every few weeks. Total treatment is about three to six months, similar to the time drug therapy requires to be effective.

Don't be afraid of ECT. It works and it's safe, even if you've had a recent heart attack, or have poorly controlled high blood pressure, or almost any other illness.

How to Deal with the Side Effects of Antidepressants

There's a little poison in every medication. However, sometimes one has to grin and bear the side effects of a drug for the greater benefit it confers. Here are some of the problems that can be caused by antidepressants—and how to deal with them:

• **Dry mouth** is possibly the most common side effect of virtually all the antidepressants. Unless you're in heart failure, you should drink as much water as you need to quench your thirst. If necessary, chew sugarless gum to stimulate the production of saliva in your mouth. Since a dry mouth predisposes cavity formation, gum infection, and tooth loss, rinse your mouth twice a day with a fluoride preparation and see your dentist three or four times a year for oral hygiene.

• **Constipation** is another common complication of antidepressants. It can be prevented by eating bran cereals every morning, drinking at least six 8-ounce glasses of water daily, eating salad twice a day, and exercising at least thirty minutes three or four times a week. Also, take a bulk-forming agent such as psyllium (Metamucil) to make your stools easier to pass. But whatever you do, don't fall into the laxative trap.

• **Bladder problems.** If you have a large prostate, the tricyclic drugs can interfere with the flow of urine out of your bladder. If it takes you longer than five minutes to get things going after you arrive at the urinal, tell your doctor about it.

• **Blurred vision** is a common side effect of the tricyclics. Chances are they won't affect your distant vision, but you may have trouble reading. Most people adjust in a few weeks, but if you don't and are apt to need these drugs for any length of time, have your glasses changed.

• **Dizziness** is another complication of the tricyclics. (Do you see now why they're not my first choice?) This symptom worries me because it can lead to a fall and serious injury. If it persists, you'll have to stop taking the drug. While using tricyclics, change position slowly to avoid a drop in blood pressure (doctors call it "orthostatic hypotension") when going from sitting to standing, or when getting out of bed. Also, make sure you're consuming enough salt and fluids.

• **Drowsiness** is frequently produced by virtually every antidepressant, though less so with the newer SSRIs. Most people adapt to it in time, and it's rarely a reason to quit taking the medication. However, while you're adjusting, don't drive or operate dangerous equipment. An extra cup of coffee will often perk you up.

• **Loss of libido** is a common side effect of the SSRIs. That's often hard to evaluate in someone who's depressed, since lack of interest in sex often accompanies depression anyway. But if it's a real problem, ask your doctor about some of the new sex medications, such as sildenafil (Viagra). And if they don't work, there's always golf.

Treatment for depression is rarely a one-shot affair. Most cases, especially among the elderly, are chronic and tend to recur, so therapy needs to be ongoing. Although drugs are the mainstay, other steps should also be taken when possible. A caring family, an understanding primary-care doctor, a skilled social worker, and self-help groups can all help implement changes in the environment and lifestyle that will ease the sadness and hopelessness that many of these people feel. But paramount in the management of depression is the treatment of any underlying disease whose symptoms are contributing to the depression.

What to Remember about Depression

1. Depression is a serious problem, especially among the elderly.
2. Depression is not an inevitable part of the aging process, but is usually due to a combination of factors—personal, environmental, and medical—acting together to produce prolonged despair.
3. Sadness is an appropriate reaction to bereavement, financial and personal problems, the realization that life is finite, and the symptoms of serious disease. But sadness becomes depression when it continues

for weeks or months and interferes with everyday living.

4. Several diseases such as Parkinson's and hypothyroidism are sometimes mistaken for depression. Every depressed person should have a pertinent physical and neurological examination to exclude these and other causes.

5. Several medications, especially those used to treat high blood pressure, can cause depression.

6. New antidepressant drugs can control depression with minimal side effects. The first choice for the elderly should be the selective serotonin reuptake inhibitors (SSRIs) such as Zoloft, Paxil, and Prozac.

7. Electroconvulsive therapy (ECT) is an effective, safe treatment for depressed persons who have not responded to antidepressants.

5

HEARING LOSS

"Nice watch. What kind is it?"
"Three o'clock."

You've just run into an old army buddy at a cocktail party. While you're reminiscing together, his wife ambles over and joins in the conversation. The last time you met them, she had no problem with her speech; but now she mumbles so badly you don't understand a word she's saying. You know that it's not your hearing because although the room is crowded and noisy, you can make out most of what her husband is saying. His voice is softer than it used to be, but then we're all getting older.

A few weeks later, you come across another woman who also can't enunciate clearly. You begin to wonder about the acoustics in these new homes. It hasn't occurred to you that you're a little deaf.

If this scenario, or any of the others described below,

are familiar to you, you're probably one of the 30 million Americans, 9 million of whom are over sixty-five, with impaired hearing. That last number is growing rapidly as life expectancy continues to increase in this country. Thirty percent of those between sixty-five and seventy years old, and 40 percent of persons older than seventy-five, have significant hearing loss.

What Causes Hearing Loss?

There are several different causes of deafness at every stage of life. Infants may be born deaf because of a congenital abnormality, faulty genetics, or some problem the mother had during pregnancy. The ears or another part of the hearing mechanism can be injured by loud noise, infections (especially of the middle and inner ear), tumors, and toxic drugs, particularly antibiotics such as streptomycin, neomycin, kanamycin, and gentamicin. (If you're taking one of these medications and notice a loss of hearing, or develop noises in your head [tinnitus, see Chapter 17] notify your doctor immediately.) If you have a serious infection that's responsive to only one of these agents and you must continue to take it despite the troublesome side effects, there's some recent good news. Researchers at the University of Michigan prevented deafness in guinea pigs taking these antibiotics by re-treating them with iron-chelating drugs that soak up extra iron in the bloodstream. Clinical trials of these chelating agents are currently underway in humans.

Deafness may also be due to some problem in the brain, so that it becomes unable to interpret the information it receives from the ears. Persons so affected hear what's said but don't understand it.

But age-related hearing loss is a special kind. You don't hear the high tones—women's voices, telephones, anything that beeps, and, for you nature lovers, the chirping birds. This selective deafness is due to a combination of degenerative changes in different parts of the ear: The ear drum is less elastic and doesn't vibrate as well when sound waves strike it; the three small bones in the middle ear that normally transmit these vibrations to the inner ear don't move as well; and, most important, little hair cells in the cochlea begin to malfunction. The cochlea is a coiled tube shaped like a snail and filled with fluid that's located in the inner ear. When its hairs move in response to sound or vibrations, they generate nerve impulses that are transmitted via the main hearing (auditory) nerve to the brain, which then interprets them as meaningful sounds.

When to Treat Your Hearing Loss

Hearing loss associated with aging can seriously affect the quality of your life. There's no way to prevent this form of deafness, except perhaps to avoid chronic exposure to loud noise. Some doctors claim, but have been unable to prove, that a low-fat diet is preventive.

The only way to treat deafness is with a hearing aid or

some other amplifying device. For some reason, many people refuse to admit that their hearing is impaired, and won't do anything about it. The following account is typical. Does it ring a bell (and can you hear it)?

You and your wife are at the theater. You've been told it's a great play and a wonderful cast. You settle back to enjoy it, but there's a problem: You can make out most of what the men are saying, but the women are mumbling. You ask your wife whether she can hear the ladies. "Of course. Can't you?" At intermission, she comes back with a headset that she rented for you in the lobby. "Try this," she says. You look around and see quite a few other people wearing them, so you put the headset on. You're amazed to find that every word spoken by both the male and female actors is now crystal clear. Even the men's voices, which you thought you were hearing perfectly well, are much more vibrant.

If this scenario is familiar to you, you may as well face the fact that you're hard of hearing. (The word *deaf* is offensive to you and probably not in your vocabulary.) If you're honest with yourself, you'll admit that you've been denying and ignoring so many things in recent months or years: You've been unfairly badgering your wife to stop mumbling; you've been sullen and frustrated because you can't hear everything that's going on around you; you don't always hear the phone ring unless you're right beside it, and when you do answer it, you often have to ask the person at the other end to speak more loudly and repeat what they've said; you find yourself looking at people's lips when they're talking to you and you can't distinguish "s," "sh," "v," "f," "t," and "b" from each other. All of this is proof that you're hard of hearing.

What are you going to do about it? Headphones to watch TV at home and at the theater and an amplifier for your phone will help. But that still leaves you unable to understand what people are saying to you at work and socially. There are no pills, diets, or exercises that will improve your hearing. Your only option is a hearing aid.

To prove that you need one, try the twenty-five-decibel rub. Find a quiet room. Extend your arm out to the side and lightly rub your thumb and forefinger together. As you do so, move them toward your ear and see at what distance you begin to hear the rubbing sound. You should be able to do so six to eight inches away. If you can't hear it at four inches, consult a hearing specialist. He or she will first look into your ears to make sure that the canals are not blocked by wax. (You'd be surprised how many "deaf" people are cured after a good ear cleaning.) When the doctor tests your hearing, she will almost certainly find that you don't hear the high frequencies in one or both ears. This condition is called presbycusis (from the Greek *presbus,* meaning "old man," and *acusis,* for "hearing.") You'll then be offered a tiny hearing aid that fits deep down into your ear canal and is visible to someone only when they actually look directly into it at very close range. You're reassured that your hearing loss can remain your secret. You're amazed that such a small hearing aid can solve your problem. However, when deafness is severe, or the problem is in the brain and not the ear, much larger devices that are very obvious are needed.

The Price of Good Hearing

You'd better sit down before you ask the audiologist what these wonderful little hearing aids will cost you. It's well over five thousand dollars for the pair. (Some lucky people only need one hearing aid, at least for a while.) "Isn't there anything less expensive?" you ask. "After all, they're so small—and they're not made of gold or diamonds, are they?" Well, you'll be told there are less expensive models but that they don't usually work as well as these digital ones (which are so expensive because they're new; I expect their price will come down in a year or two).

If you can't ante up the four or five thousand dollars, you'll just have to go on being deaf. In the United States virtually no third-party payer, whether it's Medicare, managed-care companies, private insurers, or the health plan provided by your employer, will reimburse you for them. All these "providers" consider hearing aids to be a luxury, not a necessity like, say, a new heart valve. The National Health Service in England does pay for hearing aids, as do government health plans in several other countries. It's an outrage that in this, the richest country on earth, older people of limited means who cannot afford the cost of hearing aids (or dentures, or eyeglasses) are doomed to endure deafness (as well as vision loss and the inability to chew their food).

Five or ten years ago, hearing aids were much larger than they are today—and very obvious. They whistled; they distorted sounds; they amplified every noise that hit the eardrum. At a restaurant, they gave the clatter of the dishes the same priority as tender little nothings whispered in your ear. In short, they were unable to discriminate one sound from another. Many users preferred silence to the din and refused to wear their hearing aids. Today's units are much more sophisticated. Not only are they unobtrusive (manufacturers call them "invisible"), they also reduce unwanted background noise and over-amplification. Most important, they can be programmed for different listening situations—when you're conversing with someone in a quiet room, are at a concert or the theater, watching TV, or talking on the phone. Mind you, they're by no means perfect, despite the five-thousand-dollar tab. However, you take very little chance when you order them. Most audiologists and manufacturers let you try them for up to a month and will give you your money back if you're not satisfied. But here's a word of caution: These hearing aids come with tiny batteries that have to be inserted into an equally small hinged holder on the unit. Putting them in requires a certain amount of coordination. If your hands shake or you don't see too well, you may have trouble with them. So before you commit yourself to buying or even trying these hearing aids, ask the audiologist to show you a sample pair and see if you can cope with the batteries.

Hearing aids don't do nearly as much for hearing as proper glasses or cataract surgery do for vision. You won't ever hear like you did when you were twenty. There will still be times when "f" still sounds like "s," and you will occasionally need to ask someone to repeat or clarify a remark. However, you will be able to make out more of what is said to you, even by women at cocktail parties. You'll also be able to carry on a conversation with your grand-children; you'll discover, to your delight, that the birds have not stopped chirping in your garden. (President Clinton, who has a high-frequency hearing loss, was fitted with hearing aids at age fifty-one because, according to his press secretary, "He has trouble hearing people at receptions and often can't make out what hecklers shout at him. He will wear it only when he needs it." Now there's a President for you. Imagine getting hearing aids in order to hear his heck-lers!) All in all, your life will be richer, and you'll be per-ceived as younger, not older, when your hearing aid allows you to be your old dynamic self again—even if it does oc-casionally whistle when you chew.

What to Remember about Hearing Loss

1. The hearing loss of aging (presbycusis) is fairly typ-ical and predictable. You have trouble hearing con-sonants, and you can't make out high-frequency sounds such as women's voices, phones, and other bells, especially in noisy areas.
2. There is no way to prevent or treat this form of deaf-ness, although you should always try to avoid very loud noises.
3. Presbycusis affects men more often than women; the process starts in the fifties and its progress is relent-less and insidious.

4. Hearing aids should be no more of a stigma than are gray hair, eyeglasses, or false teeth. You wear glasses because you want to be able to see; you have dentures or implants because you want to chew. There's no reason to deny your hearing loss or rationalize your deafness by refusing to do the only thing that will help matters—getting a properly fitted hearing aid.

5. Going through the later years unable to hear what's being said is an important cause of depression and withdrawal among those so affected, and often results in personal and social problems at home and at work.

6. Newer hearing aids go a long way toward solving the problem. Many are now virtually invisible (if that's important to you) and can be programmed to eliminate most of the problems associated with earlier devices.

7. When you surrender to the right hearing aid, selected and fitted by a competent audiologist, you'll enjoy victory in your fight to maintain the quality of life as you grow older.

6

HEART ATTACKS

A Preventable Epidemic

Heart attacks are the number-one killer in every developed nation (with the notable exception of Japan, where stroke has that dubious honor). Heart attacks account for more than half the deaths in the United States, where they strike 1 1/2 million people every year. Of the more than 500,000 who die from heart attacks, some 300,000 never even make it to the hospital.

A bad heart can kill at any age, but heart attacks are the major nemesis later in life; the older you are, the greater the risk.

The following true accounts are examples of some of the more important points I have tried to make in this chapter on heart attack.

Back in the early 1940s, long before I entered medical school or even thought of becoming a doctor, I knew a man, then in his middle forties, who for years had chest pain on exertion. His doctor told him it was due to indigestion and there was nothing to worry about. He never had an ECG because in those days electrocardiography was in its infancy and few general practitioners had a machine or knew how to interpret the tracing. Only heart specialists, whom few working-class people could afford to go to, took electrocardiograms in those days. This man smoked (at the time, no one, not even the surgeon general, thought it was harmful), he ate whatever he wanted (the importance of diet was not appreciated, and cholesterol was not yet a household word), and his blood pressure was a little high but never treated (few doctors believed that an elevated pressure was bad for you unless it caused symptoms).

After several years of living with "stomach" pain, this man suffered a heart attack. He remained in the hospital for six weeks, mostly at complete bed rest. When he returned home, he was told he could never work again—and he was not yet fifty years old. In the following years, his chest pain recurred frequently, and he was given the same nitroglycerin he'd been taking right along. Aspirin was only for headaches, and blood thinners were not yet being used. Heart surgery was only for a few infants born with a hole in the heart or other congenital malformations, and angiograms were still a generation away. So this man lived the rest of his life slipping nitroglycerin tablets under his tongue whenever he felt pressure in his chest. However, he was not deterred from working, because he had a son to put through medical school. Although he lived for several more years, his frequent pains reduced the quality of his life. The man was my father.

My sadness and frustration over his suffering influenced my decision to become a doctor, and especially a cardiologist, hoping to be able to help him in some way. And I could have, had he lived long enough. In the rest of this chapter you will read what I would now do for my father were I able to turn back the clock.

But first let me tell you about Mr. Jack Paar, the famous TV personality from the 1960s. One night, a few years ago, he was awakened by chest pressure that he was *almost* certain was due to indigestion. However, he had just read the chapter on heart attack in my book *Symptoms*. He awakened his wife and said to her, in effect, "I know this sounds ridiculous. I'm sure that what I'm feeling is nothing more than indigestion. I doubt that it's my heart because I've never had heart trouble before. Still, I read a book this afternoon that described my exact symptoms as being typical of a heart attack. The doctor who wrote it said to get to the hospital immediately because if it is, in fact, a heart attack, emergency treatment can save your life. What do you think we should do?" Without hesitation, she agreed to go to the nearest hospital, where his suspicions were later confirmed. He was, indeed, in the midst of an acute myocardial infarction (that's what doctors call a heart attack). He received the thrombolytic therapy described below, and he ended up without any significant cardiac muscle damage. Fifty years after my father's heart attack, which was managed by scientific inertia, Mr. Paar was spared a heart attack and restored to an active life.

These examples indicate why what you will read in the following pages is so essential to your continued good health and survival.

Arteriosclerosis: The Basic Cause

Three coronary arteries and their branches course through the heart muscle to deliver the blood and other nutrients necessary to keep it pumping. Early in life, fatty deposits begin to form on the interior lining of these vessels, a process called arteriosclerosis ("hardening of the arteries"). As we age, these fatty streaks form plaques that get progressively larger. At some point, they reduce the size of the interior diameter (lumen) of the arteries, so that less blood flows through them to supply the heart. Arteriosclerosis worsens with the years, and at age fifty becomes a potential threat to everyone. But you can hold it in check, and slow its process, as the years go by.

Risk Factors for Hardening of the Arteries—And How to Control Them

How can we prevent these plaques from forming, enlarging, and ultimately blocking our coronaries? Although we really don't understand the basic mechanism(s) involved, there are several risk factors whose presence increases vulnerability to a heart attack and, conversely, whose control or elimination is protective. The importance of any one of these risk factors is unpredictable in any given individual. Some of us appear to be resistant to their ill effects; others are not. We all know people who smoke, are overweight, have untreated high blood pressure, never exercise, and still reach a ripe old age. But take it from me, they're a very small minority. Every one of these risk factors, singly and especially in combination, leaves you vulnerable to narrowing and occlusion of the coronary arteries—and to a heart attack.

We find arteriosclerotic changes even in the arteries of children who have one or more of these risk factors. In a recent study of ninety-three individuals ages two to thirty-nine who died from a variety of noncardiac causes, only 1 percent of those without any risk factors had fatty deposits in their coronary arteries; they were present in 3 percent of those with two risk factors; in subjects with three risk factors, 8 percent had diseased coronary arteries; and 11 percent of those with four risk factors had some arterial plaque formation. So it behooves you to do your best, throughout your life, to eliminate as many risk factors as you can—and the sooner you do so, the better.

Let's take a closer look at some of the individual risk factors in the arteriosclerosis saga and see what you can do about them. They include tobacco, high blood pressure, obesity, diabetes, and blood fats, such as cholesterol and triglycerides, that are probably the greatest culprits. So let's deal with them first.

THE BLOOD FATS

• **Cholesterol** has two main components: a "good" fraction called high-density lipoprotein (HDL), and a "bad" one, low-density lipoprotein (LDL). Both HDL and LDL are attached to the cholesterol molecule. The difference between them, and the reason one is "good" and the other "bad," is that HDL carries cholesterol out of the bloodstream and away from the arterial wall (like a boat picking up passengers from the dock, in this case, the arterial wall) and deposits it in the liver (which then excretes it). LDL, on the other hand, discharges the passengers (cholesterol) onto the lining of the coronary arteries, where it eventually forms plaques. So whenever you have your cholesterol tested, make sure that the doctor also measures the HDL and LDL. According to the National Cholesterol Education Program, the ideal ratio between the total cholesterol and HDL is less than 4.5 and the LDL levels should not be higher than 130 milligrams. In my own practice, I aim for a cholesterol-to-HDL ratio of less than 4 (the lower the better), and an LDL reading below 100, especially in patients with coronary artery disease. Diet and/or drugs are the best way to lower the bad LDL; thirty minutes of aerobic exercise three or four times a week is an effective, natural way to raise your HDL.

• **Triglyceride** (cholesterol's less famous cousin) levels are also an independent risk factor. In other words, regardless of what the other blood fats are doing, a high triglyceride alone is bad news and should be corrected. Triglycerides are made in the liver; their normal range is up to 200 milligrams. However, before deciding that yours is too high, make sure that the blood is drawn after you have been fasting for at least fourteen hours. (Cholesterol may be tested at any time, regardless of what and when you last ate.)

Cholesterol is a white, waxy fat that occurs naturally in the body and is vital to your health, despite its bad reputation. Every cell needs some to build its walls and to produce certain body chemicals, such as hormones, without which we couldn't function normally. But don't rush out for a high-cholesterol meal. Your liver makes all the cholesterol you need. You'd never be lacking in it even if you had none whatsoever in your diet.

How did we come to implicate cholesterol in the causation of arteriosclerosis? Why didn't we suspect copper, zinc, magnesium, or any one of the hundreds of other body chemicals? The tip-off was the observation that the plaques within the coronary arteries are composed mainly of cholesterol and other blood fats. Several blood components involved in the clotting process are also present: platelets, fibrin, and others. That's the reason, as you will see below, that heart-attack prevention strategies deal with these substances as well as with cholesterol.

Once we determined that the plaques were rich in cholesterol, the next step was to prove that lowering its concentration in the bloodstream made a difference in a person's health. It took years to obtain that evidence, and it was acquired in stages. Cardiologists made the first breakthrough some fifteen years ago when they showed that normalizing the elevated cholesterol level *in persons who had already sustained heart attacks* reduces the number of recurrences. Subsequent research then established that normalizing high cholesterol levels in men *who do not yet have evidence of heart disease* reduces their risk for a first heart attack. The final and most recent episode in the cholesterol story was the observation that lowering cholesterol in *apparently healthy persons whose levels are "normal" and who are not especially at risk* is also beneficial, dropping the subsequent incidence of heart attacks by 37 percent in men and a whopping 57 percent in women! The implication of these latest findings is that, as is true for blood pressure, there is no such thing as a "normal" cholesterol level. The more you can lower it, either by diet, drugs, or a combination of the two, the better off you are.

What cholesterol level should you aim for? Most doctors are satisfied with less than 200 milligrams percent at any age over thirty, and no higher than 180 milligrams below age thirty. But remember too that the all important ratio of cholesterol to HDL, which should be as low as possible, and certainly no higher than 4.5.

Reducing Cholesterol by Diet

If your doctor has decided that your lipid (blood fat) profile is abnormal and needs to be treated, try altering your diet before committing yourself to medication. If you already have evidence of heart disease, follow the diet by all means, but also start on one of the lipid-lowering drugs. Once you begin taking such a drug, you'll probably need it for the rest of your life. If you discontinue it after it has normalized your cholesterol, the levels will almost certainly bounce back.

Only a third of the cholesterol in your blood comes from cholesterol-rich foods; the rest is derived from saturated fat, which the body converts to bad LDL. The key to lowering cholesterol by diet is the avoidance of foods that contain it, as well as saturated fats. Saturated fats, usually of animal origin, are bigger villains than cholesterol. So here are some basic diet tips to help you avoid these fats: Reduce your intake of red meat, bacon, sausage, hamburgers, fat in any form, organs such as liver, kidney, or brain, and dairy products. You may have all the egg whites you want, and if you really love them, you're okay eating three or four eggs a week. (Although egg yolk is rich in cholesterol, it contains very little saturated fat.) The milk you drink should be skim or low-fat; eat cheese and ice cream made from skim milk or tofu. Commercially baked products are almost always made with the whole egg unless otherwise specified. If you bake your own cakes, discard the yolk and use only the egg white.

You'll also find saturated fat in cholesterol-free nonanimal sources such as coconut oil, palm oil, and palm kernel oil. They are present in nondairy "cream substitutes," snack foods, some frozen yogurt, and other frozen desserts. Look carefully at the labels of any of these products, and don't buy any that contain those saturated oils. Corn, cotton, and soybean oils are not harmful unless they've become saturated by a process called hydrogenation when being made into margarine. This hardens them to assure a longer shelf life. So eat only "soft" or "tub" margarine, not the solid products.

Instead of the high-cholesterol, high-fat no-nos, you should focus on foods of plant origin—fruits and vegetables—as well as fish, poultry (without the skin), and veal. Foods that were formerly forbidden—shrimp, lobster, scallops, clams, crabs, and oysters—are now cleared for consumption because even though they're rich in cholesterol, they contain so little saturated fat that reasonable amounts won't do you any harm. Eat all the oysters (Who knows? They may reduce your need for Viagra) and clams you like, but limit the other shellfish to nine ounces a day.

Meat and poultry should be (and look) lean—all muscle, without visible fat. Marbled meat, in which the fat is evenly distributed, does make for a juicy and tender steak, but it's especially bad for you. If you're a hamburger lover, use only lean round and not the fat-rich regular ground.

How you prepare your food is also important. Do all your cooking and baking with vegetable oils such as canola, sunflower, corn, soybean, and olive oil; barbecue, pan-broil, and oven-broil meat, fish, and poultry dishes. When roasting or baking meat, use a rack that allows the fat to drain off. (If you find that the fat-free meat is too dry, add gravy from which the fat has been removed. To do that, refrigerate what drips off the meat; this hardens and separates the fat. If there isn't enough left over, you may add vegetable oil, one ounce to every three ounces of meat).

There's no use depriving yourself of these high-cholesterol, high-fat foods if you continue to eat potato chips, corn chips, and cheese crackers. Try to develop a taste for pretzels, air-popped popcorn, and fruit. Prepare your own sweet rolls, pancakes, waffles, and French toast; you can bet your sweet life that the commercial stuff is full of all the things you shouldn't be eating. Graham crackers and such breads as whole wheat, pumpernickel, rye, Italian, oatmeal, and raisin, as well as English muffins, are also permissible.

Many of my patients also take garlic in various forms (most commonly in "odorless" capsules) in order to lower their cholesterol (and to reduce blood pressure, prevent blood clotting, and stimulate the immune system). Over the years, various studies have concluded that garlic has modest but definite lipid-lowering properties. More recently, however, there have been several reports refuting these claims and concluding that garlic has no effect whatsoever on cholesterol levels. So eat it to enhance the flavor of your food, but garlic may not do anything for your lipid profile.

If both your cholesterol *and* triglyceride levels are high, you'll have to modify your diet in yet another way. Cut down not only on saturated fat and cholesterol, but also on carbohydrates, that is, sugars and starches. Say good-bye to most desserts and sweets, and drink no more than 1 ounce of hard liquor, 2 1/2 ounces of dry table wine, or 4 1/2 ounces of beer per day. You may still eat all the vegetables you want, but limit your fruit intake to one serving or a half-cup of any fresh, unsweetened variety. You may still have gelatin (ugh), angel food cake, or sugar-free fruit ice. (Remember, also, that exercise and weight loss are particularly effective in lowering an elevated triglyceride level.)

As you deprive yourself of so many foods that give you pleasure, take heart in the knowledge that your new diet will probably prolong your life and spare you misery down the line. It's only fair to remind you, however, that people with normal, even low cholesterol readings can develop blocked arteries. That's important to know so that you won't ignore the other risk factors just because you're being good about your diet.

If you've followed a rigorous, low-cholesterol diet as best you can but find either that you can't continue it indefinitely or that your cholesterol has not dropped by 20 to 30 percent, it's time to think about the medication alternative. Don't have a guilty conscience about it, either, because the chance of dropping your cholesterol to optimal levels with diet alone is not great. First of all, it will only really work if you also engage in a regular exercise program. And the truth is that diet alone is effect in probably no more than 5 or 6 percent of patients.

Cholesterol-Lowering Drugs

Medications formerly used to lower cholesterol were either ineffective or caused unpleasant side effects. The introduction of the statin family of drugs has changed all that. These agents, of which there are six at the time of this writing, with more on the way, lower total cholesterol, raise the "good" HDL, and decrease the "bad"

LDL. They do so painlessly, safely, effectively—and expensively. However, like every medication, they sometimes produce side effects (muscle cramping and injury, as well as liver damage), which almost always clear up when the drug is stopped.

The liver contains receptor cells that remove cholesterol molecules from the blood as it flows through the organ. They then bind them so that the liver can later excrete them into the bowel and out of the body. That's much better than having them remain in the bloodstream, which means they can be deposited in the walls of your arteries, ultimately blocking them. The statin drugs block the enzyme that prevents the liver from making these receptor cells.

The statin drugs lower cholesterol, shrink the plaques in people who already have them, reduce the incidence of future heart attacks and strokes by lowering the LDL and raising the HDL, decrease the death rate from heart disease, and reduce overall mortality. They also act on the plaques in such a way as to lessen the chance of their rupturing and suddenly occluding a coronary artery to cause a heart attack. That's quite a list of accomplishments.

Given all these proven beneficial effects and since the sooner you reduce a high cholesterol level the better, it makes no sense for doctors to continue withholding these drugs while continuing to cajole recalcitrant patients who are vulnerable to heart disease about their diet. This simply allows the plaques to form and enlarge while the frustrated patients "try" to comply. That's why, although I continue to encourage a prudent diet, I also prescribe a statin drug to virtually every adult at risk.

If the statins aren't effective in your case, or have side effects that preclude your taking them, there are other medications that can do the job. These include gemfibrozil (Lopid), cholestyramine (Questran), and nicotinic acid (this is *niacin,* which has nothing to do with *nicotine*). They all work on the liver in different ways to reduce your cholesterol level. Although they are effective, I use them as second-line drugs after the statins because I have found them to be not quite as effective.

A question does remain: Should people in their seventies and eighties who are otherwise well but whose cholesterol level is high start dieting and/or take a statin drug? The data are conflicting. Some studies conclude that, like quitting smoking, you're never too old to "eat right"; others say leave well enough alone and don't alter a lifestyle that has a good track record. According to one recent report, persons older than seventy-five actually fare better when their cholesterol is high. Nonetheless, I continue to advise everyone to eat a low-fat, low-cholesterol diet, but I don't insist that they be compulsive about it. For example, if a perfectly healthy elderly patient with a cholesterol, say, of 240, who has never paid any attention to diet, asks for my advice, I tell him or her not to change a thing. They, their genes, or their bodies must be doing something right. I normally prescribe medication to lower cholesterol only for seniors who've had a heart attack.

Some Unanswered Questions

Exciting as they are, these new research data have raised several important questions that remain unanswered. How early in life is it safe to start anticholesterol medication, and how long should it be continued? What are its long-term effects on the growth and development of youngsters? Although they lower cholesterol, might these agents, many years down the line, hurt the immune system or increase the likelihood of cancer? Is it wise to give any drug to anyone, at any age, for a lifetime?

Several studies suggest that "abnormally" low cholesterol readings (I interpret that as under 140) are associated with a higher incidence of violent deaths—accidents, suicides, and homicides. These findings were originally dismissed as spurious and mere statistical artifacts. However, these observations keep cropping up in some studies (though not in others). Some researchers still believe that there is an association between very low cholesterol and violent behavior, but they aren't sure why. I'm keeping an open mind on the subject.

Monkeys and rats in whom cholesterol levels are lowered become more aggressive, presumably because the serotonin levels in the brain are reduced. Serotonin plays an important role in human behavior. The most widely used psychotropic drugs, the selective serotonin reuptake inhibitors (SSRIs) such as Prozac, calm you down and make you happy by *raising* the serotonin content.

How should we act on these observations? Until some of these seminal questions are answered, it's hard to be sure. I do not prescribe the statin drugs until the late teens or early twenties (and I do not recommend a diet low in saturated fat and cholesterol until after age two), except in those rare cases with a severe familial cholesterol disorder that causes heart attacks in childhood.

TOBACCO, HIGH BLOOD PRESSURE, DIABETES, AND OBESITY

• **Tobacco** is also a major risk factor for heart attacks because it accelerates arteriosclerosis. Most people think smoking is bad mainly because it causes lung cancer. They're right: It does lead to lung cancer. However, in terms of sheer numbers, most of the 350,000 deaths caused by tobacco every year in this country are the result of vascular disease and heart attacks.

You'll never hear any debate about tobacco like you do about cholesterol. No one has ever suggested that too little tobacco may be harmful. The universally agreed-upon target for the number of cigarettes you should smoke is an unequivocal zero. However, the world is full of people who pay no attention to any risk factors for heart disease. Winston Churchill is their role model. He did everything that was bad for his health—he drank, smoked, was overweight, and lived through the stress of fighting and winning wars—yet he lived into his nineties. But the exception does not prove the rule.

It's never too late to benefit from quitting tobacco. Between two to five years after you do, you eliminate your increased chances of having a heart attack. Even if you're elderly and think you've escaped the ravages of tobacco, you're always vulnerable to it. Nicotine throws arteries everywhere into temporary spasm with each puff you take. Plaques already in your coronaries—and we all have them—can shut down the arteries briefly after just one cigarette.

The first requirement for breaking the tobacco habit is a genuine wish to do so, and it must be more than lip service. Most people have the necessary motivation only after they've developed cancer or suffered a heart attack. Don't wait for that. If you can't stop "cold turkey" (which is what most ex-smokers have done), there are available aids. Some addicts are helped by acupuncture, others by hypnosis. The success rate of these interventions isn't high, but they do work occasionally. Some doctors report a 30 percent abstinence rate for one year using nicotine patches that release small amounts of the drug through the skin. Nicotine gum appears to be less effective, and some of my patients have become addicted to it. Buproprion, an anti-anxiety agent marketed as Zyban, can also help. They're all worth a try.

When you finally do stop smoking, you'll probably have nicotine withdrawal symptoms for about two weeks. You'll be irritable, nervous, impossible to live with, tired, lethargic, even light-headed—and hungry, oh so hungry!

Here's what to do: Get plenty of exercise—walk, bike, swim, do some calisthenics. That'll help you stop thinking about the missing weed. You can satisfy your hunger with lots of raw vegetables and starches, but no saturated fats or refined sugar; and drink as much water as you can. Stay determined. Eventually, you won't miss cigarettes one bit, and, like me, you may even end up complaining about the smell when someone near you lights up.

• **High blood pressure** is another very important risk factor for arteriosclerosis. However, unlike tobacco addiction, it's easily treatable. Although some people with long-standing hypertension, especially women, remain free of significant coronary artery disease for most of their lives, the majority do not. If you've already got heart trouble, normalizing an elevated pressure substantially reduces the risk of a heart attack—at any age. Your arteries are never immune to blood under high pressure pounding against their walls.

There is a prevalent myth that only the lower blood pressure figure, the diastolic, counts, and that the top number, the systolic, doesn't matter. That's absolutely (and dangerously) wrong. The combination of elevated systolic pressures and normal diastolic pressures is very common in older people, and is an important cause of strokes. So have your pressure monitored at regular intervals throughout life, even if it's always been normal.

We used to think that any reading below 140/90 was normal in adults. We now know that if the diastolic pressure is 80, you're at half the risk of having a heart attack than when it's 90.

Unless the systolic pressure readings are very high (well above 200) and pose an immediate risk of stroke, I hold off on medication while I try to get my patients to lose weight, reduce their sodium intake (to less than 2 grams of salt a day—that's 1 level teaspoon; the average American diet contains 4 to 5 grams of sodium), and exercise (walking briskly for twenty minutes to one hour a day three to five times a week, along with daily stretching and range-of-motion exercises). I also advise them not to drink more than three cups of coffee a day, and to stop smoking. If these measures are not successful, I then prescribe drugs. However, I do not do so for patients over the age of sixty-five whose pressure is less than 150/90. Too low a pressure in elderly persons can cause neurological and cardiac problems.

Drugs that lower high blood pressure still have a bad reputation because the older ones used to cause constipation, impotence, fatigue, and a slew of other side effects. However, they have been largely superseded by a new generation of effective and well-tolerated medications such as beta-blockers (Tenormin, Lopressor, Inderal), ACE inhibitors (Vasotec, Capoten, Altace, and several others), and calcium channel blockers (Procardia, Cardizem, verapamil). However, diuretics, the old standby, remain an important part of most regimens.

We have learned over the years that rather than increasing the dosage of one drug until it works, it's better to combine several of them in small amounts. Because of their synergistic, additive properties, they lower blood pressure more effectively when combined and with fewer side effects than does pushing any single agent. There is no longer any reason to forgo treatment for hypertension because of side effects.

• **Diabetics** who don't control their blood sugar level, who are overweight, and whose cholesterol and other blood fats are abnormal are especially prone to arteriosclerosis. So it's extremely important for every diabetic to maintain blood sugar levels as close to normal as possible, to take the necessary steps, using diet or medications, to normalize the blood lipids, and to attain and maintain ideal weight. The alternative is a premature heart attack.

• **Obesity,** defined as greater than 30 percent above ideal weight, as well as simple overweight, which is more common, are important risk factors for heart attack. Americans are the fattest people in the world, and 70 percent of patients with coronary artery disease are overweight. Being 10 percent above ideal weight raises your risk of a heart attack by 30 percent, especially if the extra pounds are in your belly, not your hips. You can determine your risk by measuring your waist at the belly button and your hips at their widest point. Divide the waist measurement by the hip measurement. Any number higher than 0.95 in men and 0.8 in women means a higher risk of heart disease.

I wish I had a sure-fire way to help you lose weight. But you can only succeed if you have an ongoing commitment to avoid high-calorie foods and to follow a daily exercise regimen. Forget diet pills—they're either ineffective after a short time or dangerous to your health. Don't be taken in by "fat-free" or "reduced-fat" foods.

The fat is usually replaced by calories from sugar. Look for hidden calories in salad dressings; use vinaigrette for salads and mustard for sandwiches; eat smaller meals more often.

Eliminating Other Risk Factors

If several of your *close blood relatives* have had heart attacks before the age of sixty, you're likely to have one too unless you eliminate all the other possible risk factors. Don't have a fatalistic view about heart disease because so many of your close relatives died young from heart attacks. Chances are your ill-fated parents or siblings smoked, were overweight, were diabetic with poor sugar control, had elevated cholesterol levels, and rarely exercised. Genes are only part of the story. Regardless of your genetic vulnerability, correcting any obvious abnormalities will improve your outlook considerably.

• **Regular exercise** that's sufficiently rigorous protects the coronary arteries. However, you've got to pay attention to the other risk factors as well. Dr. William Castelli, the director of the Framingham Heart Study, estimates that half the doctors running in the Boston Marathon have abnormal cholesterol levels—and don't know it!

You're most likely to stay with your exercise program if you enjoy it. Few people will continue for very long with a regimen that they find boring. Brisk walking for thirty minutes a day or vigorous gardening are enough. If you prefer, you may also run, jog, dance, bike, or swim, provided your doctor has cleared you to do so. Walking briskly for about three miles (you can pick any other form of exercise) was found to reduce the risk of a heart attack by 64 percent in male Harvard alumni. (Graduates of Princeton, Yale, and Cornell can probably expect the same good results.)

Aerobic exercises such as walking or running (as opposed to stretching and weight-lifting) exert their beneficial effect in several ways: They lower your resting heart rate and blood pressure, thus easing the burden on your heart; they reduce cholesterol and triglycerides, raise the good HDL and lower the bad LDL; they drop the blood sugar in diabetics; they help prevent osteoporosis; they decrease the proportion of body fat; they reduce stress and improve mood. All in all, exercise is a good prescription against heart attack.

• **Certain personality types** are said to be more prone to heart attacks, especially Type A—characteristically hard-driving, aggressive, hostile, and time-conscious. Yet many such people who live by the philosophy that "time is money" retire with fat pensions from senior executive jobs and attain ripe old age. By the same token, the noncompetitive, placid, unruffled, Type B personalities are certainly not free of or immune to arteriosclerosis. I believe that hostility and chronic anger are a greater threat to you than your personality. I feel sorry for the guy who sits on his car horn, cuts out in front of me, and curses me because he thinks I drive like a dunce. He may not make his fiftieth birthday. In one study, 15 percent of young doctors and lawyers with innate hostility were dead by age fifty. Such recurrent blowups are probably lethal because they release adrenaline, which, in turn, increases heart rate and raises blood pressure. If you're hostile, get rid of your anger by exercising instead of throwing a tantrum.

• **Various infections** have been implicated in the causation of arteriosclerosis. Researchers have demonstrated the presence of several viruses and bacteria in arteriosclerotic plaques. It has even been suggested that everyone with heart disease be screened for antibodies to chlamydia, and that those who have them be treated with the appropriate antibiotic. The majority of patients who've had heart attacks do not have these antibodies, and this is not a widely accepted theory. According to other researchers, there is an association between one particularly virulent strain of *H. pylori,* the bacterium implicated in the development of peptic ulcers (and possibly gastric cancer, too), and heart disease. Among eighty-six patients with arteriosclerotic heart disease, 62 percent were infected with *H. pylori,* as compared to an incidence of only 40 percent in a disease-free control group. Their recommendation? Anyone with ulcers who is shown to have *H. pylori* should be treated with antibiotics to kill the bug, not only for the sake of his stomach, but also for the good of his heart. Finally, there is a school of thought that believes that the cytomegalovirus is an important cause of heart attacks, and that patients with cardiac disease should be treated with the appropriate antibiotics for this virus as well.

But most people who've had heart attacks have no sign of any of these infections.

• **When a woman reaches menopause,** she becomes as vulnerable to heart attacks as a man. That's because she no longer has enough of the hormones that protected her when she was still having her periods. I discuss the management of menopause in detail in Chapter 10. However, suffice it to say here that in 1991, in the Nurses' Health Study, postmenopausal women taking estrogen for fifteen years had a 40 percent lower death rate from all causes than did those who didn't. Other studies have shown that menopausal women taking estrogen have fewer heart attacks than those who don't. According to the American Heart Association, estrogen replacement reduces the risk of heart attack by one-third to one-half. It may exert this protective effect by raising the good HDL, lowering blood pressure, and acting directly on the heart muscle and artery walls.

However, there are some new findings of which you should be aware. HRT apparently doesn't favorably alter the course of heart disease in women who already have it. Within one year of starting a combination of estrogen and progesterone (such as Prempro), women with documented heart disease are 50 percent *more* likely to have a heart attack. Two years later, however, their risk is 40 percent *lower.* That may be because estrogen promotes clotting in some women, but if you make it through the first year after the attack, then its cholesterol-lowering effect predominates. Here's how I suggest you act on this new information: If you already have heart disease, don't start on hormone replacement therapy. If you have some form of heart trouble and have been taking estrogen for more than a year, then it's probably safe to continue, especially if you're being given the hormone for some other reason, such as osteoporosis.

• **Elevated blood levels of homocysteine** have recently become suspect as a cause of arteriosclerosis, although the theory suggesting their importance goes back several years. The normal range of homocysteine is 5 to 15 micromols; in patients with coronary disease, values of 20 or more are often observed. (However, most cardiac patients have normal readings.) These high levels return to normal when supplemental folic acid is taken. I now routinely screen all my "high-risk" adult patients for homocysteine and prescribe 1 to 2 milligrams of folic acid to virtually all of them. Low doses of estrogen also reduce homocysteine levels—but not many men will accept the female hormones!

• **Several studies have suggested that excess iron increases the risk of heart disease.** In one large Finnish study, those with the least ferritin (the protein that carries iron) in the blood are said to develop 50 percent fewer heart attacks. The explanation given is that iron facilitates the formation of plaques by LDL. The researchers postulate that premenopausal women are usually free from heart disease, not necessarily or solely because of their female hormones, but because they lose iron when they bleed every month. This interesting theory needs confirmation. In the meantime, there's no point in taking extra iron if you don't need it. If you're on a multivitamin supplement, check the label to see whether it contains iron. Many of them do.

Sudden Cardiac Death

Among the 1 million heart attacks in the United States every year, more than 300,000 are "sudden"—that is, abrupt and without warning; the patient either dies instantaneously or within a few hours. People who die in this way are not free of disease right up to the moment of the acute, catastrophic event. Most of them have had some earlier warning; many either didn't recognize the signals or denied them and did nothing about them. However, there are some individuals in whom heart disease is "silent," especially diabetics, whose nervous system is affected by their disease so that it doesn't transmit pain sensation. Their fatal attacks happen out of the blue. That's why routine cardiac diagnostic tests to detect silent heart disease (described later in this chapter) are so important for everyone who's vulnerable.

Symptoms of Heart Trouble

What are the symptoms of heart trouble? How can you be sure that what you're experiencing isn't due to something else, like indigestion or some other disorder?

A small amount of plaque here and there in an artery is no cause for alarm; every "healthy" person has them. Plaque deposits do not cause symptoms until they reduce the amount of blood flow below a critical level. You'll know that's happened when you feel *pressure or pain in your chest* after some activity that challenges your heart, such as walking quickly (especially uphill, in cold weather, or after eating), experiencing severe emotional stress, or lying down. This symptom is called *angina pectoris* (a Latin term, *angina* means "pain," *pectoris* is "chest").

Angina results from any demand on the heart that makes it work harder, so that it needs more blood. When the coronary arteries are significantly narrowed they cannot provide that extra blood. The pressure in your chest (usually behind the breastbone), is your heart's warning to stop what you're doing because it can't keep up with you. It's a cry for more oxygen. The greater the degree of arterial obstruction and the larger the blood vessel, the less exertion it takes to provoke angina. Simply going to bed also means more work for the heart. When you're standing or sitting, blood is kept in your legs and belly by the pull of gravity; when you lie down, it flows back to the heart. The heart then must work harder to expel this increased volume with each contraction. If your arteries are clogged and can't provide the additional blood, you'll have angina. Nocturnal angina usually indicates advanced disease.

I'd like to emphasize the term *chest pressure* to describe angina rather than *pain* because many people ignore cardiac symptoms that aren't "painful."

• **The major characteristic of angina** is that it clears up promptly (within a minute or two) after the activity that caused it ends—you stop walking, or end the argument, or turn off the TV with the baseball game or wrestling match that excited you, or get up from bed and sit in a chair. Nitroglycerin, in the form of a tablet or sprayed under the tongue, relieves angina within a minute or two. As you will see later, if your symptoms continue after you've stopped doing whatever caused them or the "nitro" that always relieved them in the past has no effect, they're either not angina or you may be having a heart attack.

• **The location of the chest pain or pressure** is also important. Most people wrongly believe that cardiac symptoms are felt on the left side of the chest and that's where the heart is situated. Wrong! The heart lies in the center of the chest, behind the breastbone, where you're most likely to experience angina. However, the heart's pain fibers leave the spinal cord at the same level as nerves to other nearby organs such as the chest wall, the stomach, and the lungs. So pain anywhere above the belly button may reflect either cardiac or noncardiac conditions.

• **Shortness of breath** when you're doing something that never bothered you before—walking, dancing, running, losing your temper—may also signify heart trouble. This symptom has many possible explanations: the weight you've gained, a new or worsened preexisting lung condition, or perhaps you're simply not in shape because you're a couch potato. Interestingly enough, if you're short of breath while sitting around doing nothing, it may either be very serious or of no significance whatsoever. How so? Difficulty breathing at rest, especially when lying down, may reflect congestion of the lungs due to heart failure; on the other hand, if you're unable to take a deep, satisfying breath, you may simply be hyperventilating because you're anxious.

• **Palpitations** for no apparent reason may indicate an underlying heart problem. Most of us are aware of an "extra beat" now and then, especially after drinking too much coffee, using decongestants to relieve the symptoms of a cold, or taking more thyroid replacement hormone than we need. But coronary artery disease, as well as other cardiac disorders, can also cause irregularities of cardiac rhythm, especially with exertion.

If you develop any of the symptoms described above—chest pain or pressure, shortness of breath, or palpitations—think "heart," especially if you're a man over forty or a postmenopausal woman.

How do you know for sure that these symptoms are coming from the heart? You don't, and don't try to diagnose them yourself. That's your doctor's job. The first thing he or she will (or should) do is listen carefully to their descriptions. Some doctors dispense with this "formality" and proceed directly to testing because they're pressed for time these days. Others have more confidence in machines than they do in their judgment. Both reasons are unfortunate, because a careful interview can be more revealing than any test (and cheaper, too).

In addition to listening to your account, your doctor

should review your past medical history and record in order to see whether you are especially vulnerable to arteriosclerosis. Do you have high blood pressure, diabetes, and/or a high cholesterol level? Are you a smoker? Did other members of your family have premature heart disease? However, even if you have none of these risk factors, you can still have the disease. Hospitals are full of patients who are exceptions to the rule.

Testing for Angina

Having taken a good history, your doctor proceeds to the physical exam, paying particular attention to your weight, blood pressure, heart, lungs, and eye grounds. (The back of your eye is the only part of the body where arteries are actually visible and can reveal evidence of arteriosclerosis. Everywhere else, we feel them or listen to them.) When examining your chest, the doctor listens for heart murmurs and for congestion or fluid in the lungs. The exam also focuses on the vascular system, looking for abnormalities in the circulation of your legs, neck, and abdomen.

After completing the physical exam, which may well be normal and unrevealing, it's time for some tests. Blood and urine are sent to the laboratory. The doctor is especially interested in your cholesterol and other blood fats, in your sugar level (are you diabetic?), and whether your liver and kidneys are functioning normally.

Next comes the electrocardiogram (ECG). Although this is a very useful tool, it may surprise you to learn that it is absolutely normal in about 75 percent of people with angina. If it is, and the doctor suspects angina, you'll need a stress test.

A stress test makes the heart work hard enough to require more blood. If your coronary arteries are narrowed, they cannot provide the extra supply needed. The ECG recorded during or after exercise usually becomes abnormal regardless of whether or not the stress itself has reproduced your symptoms.

There are several different kinds of stress tests. Years ago, we simply had the patient walk up and down a small staircase a prescribed number of times, depending on age and sex, and then recorded the electrocardiogram after it was completed. However, the treadmill and the stationary bicycle have largely superseded the Master Two-Step Test (developed by my late father-in-law, Dr. Arthur M. Master, and named after him).

All electrocardiographic stress tests have a certain incidence of false-negative results (the patient has heart disease but the test is normal) and false positives (the ECG becomes abnormal even though the subject is free of disease). Healthy women often have a falsely "positive" stress test and need to undergo one of the more sophisticated diagnostic procedures described below.

If the doctor suspects that your stress test is either falsely positive or falsely negative, you'll go to the next level of testing, of which there are several different types. The stress echo records an echocardiogram in addition to the ECG tracing. This provides a view of the beating heart. When the blood supply to any portion of it is inadequate after exercise, the affected area beats less vigorously—and this "sluggishness" is apparent on the echo.

There are also several expensive nuclear procedures that can be done, the best known of which is the thallium test. This compares the amount of blood delivered to the heart muscle at rest and during exercise. Other newer methods using MRIs, PET scans, and CT scans of the heart are being developed. At the present time, the thallium test is the most widely preferred of the lot.

If you have arthritis or for some other reason are unable to walk quickly enough on a treadmill or pedal on a stationary bike, you can be "stressed" at rest. This is done by injecting you with a drug that simulates exercise by increasing the work of the heart.

Treatment of Angina

If any of these examinations confirm the diagnosis of angina, you can be treated with a variety of drugs. The most important is *nitroglycerin,* which you should keep with you at all times. At the very first indication of angina, you must stop what you're doing, sit down, and put a nitro under your tongue. (If you remain standing, you may pass out because nitroglycerin widens arteries, not only in the heart, but everywhere else in the body, causing your blood pressure to drop.) Your angina will disappear in seconds or minutes. There are many long-acting nitro derivatives (Isordil, Ismo, and Imdur) that widen the coronary arteries for hours at a time. These can be either taken by mouth once or twice a day or applied topically in a cream, ointment, or patch.

There are other drugs with anti-anginal properties, such as the *calcium channel* and *beta-blockers*. I also prescribe 400 to 800 units of *vitamin E* to all my patients with coronary artery disease since there have been several studies suggesting that this antioxidant vitamin reduces the incidence of heart attacks. I also give a statin drug to lower cholesterol, regardless of its level. The key, however, is a *daily low-dose aspirin* (81 milligrams). It should be coated to reduce the risk of irritating or ulcerating the lining of your upper intestinal tract. Aspirin acts on the platelets in the blood to reduce the tendency of the coronary arteries to form clots. Low-dose aspirin reduces the risk of heart attack by almost 50 percent. (Unless there is some reason for them not to take it, I recommend a "baby" aspirin every other day to all healthy men over age forty, and to postmenopausal women. Other doctors sometimes prescribe more.)

If your coronary artery disease is mild, that is, with significant blockages in only one vessel or minimal obstruction in several, then medication alone will control your symptoms and allow you to lead a virtually normal life.

CORONARY ANGIOGRAPHY

Because severity of symptoms does not always correlate well with the extent of disease, many cardiologists encourage their patient with angina to have an *angiogram*. In this invasive procedure (none of the aforementioned stress tests are invasive), dye is injected into the coronary arteries through a catheter placed in an artery (usually in the groin, but sometimes in the forearm). You remain awake, and it's painless. If you're interested, you can even look at your coronaries on the screen as they're being studied. An angiogram permits the doctor to view the entire cardiac circulation, and to determine how many vessels are diseased, which ones, and how badly. This information tells us whether it's safe to continue treating you with medication or whether the obstructions are life-threatening and must be relieved.

BALLOON ANGIOPLASTY

If it appears, from the angiogram, that you are in danger of one of these narrowed arteries closing completely and causing a heart attack (see below), you may be advised to have an angioplasty or some other procedure to unclog the affected artery. This is often done while you're still on the table. A catheter with a tiny collapsed balloon at its tip is threaded to the obstructed area in the coronary artery, positioned alongside the blockage, and then inflated. This compresses the plaque against the vessel wall and widens its interior diameter. To make sure that the artery stays open, a metal stent (like a sleeve) is frequently placed in the ballooned area. Angioplasty has sharply reduced the need for bypass operations.

Instead of ballooning the diseased artery open, the doctor may literally scrape away the obstructing plaque (atherectomy) or, less frequently, vaporize it with a laser. In most cases, you can go home the next morning on aspirin or some other blood-thinning medication that helps prevent the treated vessel from clotting.

If the arteries seen on the angiogram are too severely or diffusely diseased to be angioplastied, your next option is bypass surgery.

THE BYPASS OPERATION

In the early 1970s, a bypass operation took twelve or more hours and carried with it a mortality rate between 5 and 10 percent. An experienced surgeon (the only kind to have) can now bypass several coronary arteries in three to four hours, at a risk of less than 1 percent.

In the bypass operation, blood is supplied by the aorta (the large vessel coming out of the heart that branches into the other major arteries in the body). One end of a healthy blood vessel, which is taken from either a large vein in the leg (saphenous) or, preferably, one of the internal mammary arteries in the chest wall, is attached to the aorta, and the other end is sewn into the coronary artery beyond the point at which it is obstructed. (That's why the operation is called a "bypass.") This operation can only be done when the caliber of the diseased coronary is sufficiently free of disease and large enough to accept the grafted vessel.

When arteriosclerosis is diffuse and involves the entire coronary artery, not just one or two discrete areas, there's no place to put the graft.

The traditional bypass operation requires the chest to be opened with an incision through the middle of the breastbone, which is then spread apart to expose the heart. Newer techniques, the minimally invasive direct coronary artery bypass (MIDCAB) procedure and the PortoCath, do not require the chest to be opened. Instead, the surgeon inserts the instruments through several small holes in the chest. At the present time, this simpler approach is usually done to repair only one of the three coronary vessels, the middle one, called the left anterior descending (LAD). However, some surgeons are performing multiple bypasses in this way, and are also even replacing heart valves without opening the chest. Several of my patients who have had these procedures were able to leave the hospital after a day or two instead of the five or more days required by more extensive operations.

When a bypass is not possible because there are no vessels of adequate size to which to attach a graft, all is not lost. There are two new approaches, still in the experimental stage, which are sometimes successful. The first is the laser revascularization procedure. The doctor threads a catheter into the interior of the heart. A laser gun at its tip is then positioned against the inside wall of the heart and directs its beams, thinner than a human hair, at the heart muscle. Since this is done from within the heart, the chest need not be opened. After a few weeks, the channels made by the laser beams form new vascular conduits in the heart muscle that eventually take over from the original blocked arteries. Some doctors prefer to deliver the laser beam through a small incision in the chest. In another, equally exciting, alternative to bypass surgery, genes that promote the formation of new blood vessels (vascular growth factor) are injected directly into the heart muscle, where they form new blood vessels that in time provide nutrition to the heart.

The Important Collaterals

Over the years, as the coronary artery plaques increase in size and progressively reduce the amount of blood delivered to the heart muscle, a protective mechanism called *collateral circulation* develops. We're all born with a network of tiny blood vessels distributed throughout the heart muscle. As the amount of available oxygen to the muscle decreases, these tiny channels dilate and eventually deliver their own blood supply to the heart muscle. Whether you live or die after a heart attack depends on several factors: the size of the occluded vessel (the larger it is, the more blood it carries, and the greater the area of the heart it supplies), the condition of your other coronaries and how well they are able to compensate for the acute blockage, how much heart muscle was affected, and, last but not least, the extent of the collateral circulation.

The Evolution of a Heart Attack

If you have angina, you are a candidate for a heart attack. The vessels that have been narrowed suddenly close, usually because an arteriosclerotic plaque has ruptured, or a fresh clot (thrombus) has formed on its surface. Whatever the cause, blood flow to the heart muscle is shut off. When that happens, the portion of the heart supplied by the obstructed vessel dies. If the affected area is large enough, you may not survive. Also, the dying cardiac muscle, with its lowered oxygen content, may trigger electrical activity that causes ventricular fibrillation, an uncoordinated twitching of the heart that leaves it unable to pump blood. Unless ventricular fibrillation is treated instantly by electrical shock, in the ambulance or in the emergency room, it is uniformly fatal. (Every suspected heart attack patient is hooked up to an ECG machine promptly after arriving at the hospital so that he or she can be treated immediately should ventricular fibrillation develop.)

Is It a Heart Attack?

The typical symptoms of a heart attack are pressure, fullness, squeezing, or pain in the center of the chest behind the breastbone. It often spreads to the arms, shoulders, through to the back, the jaw, the throat, and even the ears. These symptoms are very much like angina, which usually (but not always) precedes the heart attack for a varying period of time. However, symptoms of a heart attack are much more severe than angina, and unlike the latter, they occur at rest, not with exertion. A nitroglycerin tablet may ease the pain for a few seconds or minutes, but it returns. You may feel weak, short of breath, light-headed, faint, and/or nauseated. You may also be aware of your heartbeat or have palpitations, and chances are you'll also be in a cold sweat. Most patients are very apprehensive because they know instinctively that there is something very seriously wrong. You're apt to feel better in a sitting position than lying down. You can't see what you look like unless you're in front of a mirror, but you appear very pale and sick-looking to anyone who happens to observe you.

This is the classical presentation of a heart attack. In real life, however, no two cases are the same, and the combination of symptoms listed above may vary. If you have the slightest suspicion that you're having a heart attack, take an aspirin and get to the nearest hospital emergency room as fast as you can. Either call 911 for an ambulance or have someone drive you. Don't wait for your doctor to respond to your telephone call. Nor is this the time to be testing your diagnostic skills, wondering whether you're suffering from a stomach problem, a lung disorder, or a muscle spasm. The symptoms of heart attack may mimic several other conditions; differentiating one from the other is a doctor's job, not yours. Remember, "Time is muscle." Get to the emergency room fast.

When you tell the triage nurse in the emergency room (whose job it is to separate the sheep from the goats as far as symptoms are concerned) that you are having chest pain, you will (or should) be taken care of immediately. There's none of the protracted waiting endured by those with such trivial (by comparison) problems as pneumonia, a fracture, or a high fever. You will be seen by a doctor without delay. Someone will give you oxygen, another aide will hook you up to an electrocardiograph machine, a nurse will take your blood pressure. You will be connected to a heart monitor so that your electrocardiogram and blood pressure are displayed at all times, and a technician will start an intravenous injection so that if you require emergency drugs at any time, they can be given by vein without delay. Blood will be drawn to test whether you are "spilling enzymes" (when heart muscle is damaged by a heart attack, it releases specific enzymes that can be measured in the blood), and you will be given nitroglycerin. All this is just in case, even before they know for sure whether or not you're really having a heart attack. During these hectic (and necessary) precautions, the doctor will be performing a very focused cardiac examination. The ECG alone may not be enough to diagnose the presence of an acute heart attack because it can remain normal during the first few hours after the onset of symptoms. That's why all these other tests are done.

If the evidence points to an acute heart attack, there are several treatment options: You can be managed conservatively, that is, you are admitted to the coronary care unit of the hospital and the oxygen is continued, intravenous anticoagulants are administered along with oral aspirin to thin your blood, you're given nitroglycerin intravenously and coronary dilator drugs by mouth, you take other medications such as ACE inhibitors and/or beta-blockers to ease the strain on the threatened heart muscle, and your blood pressure is controlled (raised if it's too low, lowered if it's too high). These days, however, many heart attack patients, especially those in large medical centers, are treated more aggressively. If you arrive less than three or four hours after the onset of your symptoms, the doctor may give you one of several agents to dissolve the fresh clot that's obstructing the artery (thrombolytic therapy). This often restores some blood flow to the affected area of the heart. When such therapy works, as it often does, the electrocardiographic evidence of cardiac injury improves dramatically and your chest symptoms are relieved.

Another option is an emergency angiogram. If you're lucky, the fresh clot in the diseased artery can be opened up with a balloon and blood flow restored before there has been permanent damage to the heart muscle. So you see why it is critical to go to the hospital fast even if you only *suspect* that you're having a heart attack. It's better to be safe than sorry. Help in time can save your life and prevent permanent injury to your heart.

Occasionally, despite all the measures described above, the chest pain persists, the ECG abnormalities worsen, the cardiac enzyme levels continue to rise, and blood pressure falls to shock levels. This drastic situation may call for emergency bypass heart surgery. If it does, don't despair. Thanks to modern technology, these oper-

ations can be done safely even in the midst of an acute
heart attack.

Life after a Heart Attack

It wasn't so long ago that if you survived a heart attack,
you were expected, and indeed obliged, to retire—not
only from work, but also from life itself. Even insurance
companies, not known for their generosity or magnanim-
ity, considered such people totally disabled, regardless of
whether or not they had any symptoms after their attack.
Not only did they lose their jobs, they were also cautioned to lead a very quiet, passive, sedentary, stress-free
existence. Many became great Scrabble players and TV
aficionados.

All that's changed. The world is full of heads of state,
CEOs, practicing doctors, lawyers and other professionals, and even blue-collar workers who have returned to
their jobs and continued to lead active, normal lives. All
this has been made possible not only by successful angioplasties and coronary artery surgery, but by the host of
newer drugs that prevent recurrences, minimize symptoms, strengthen the heart muscle, control chronic disturbances of heart rhythm, keep the coronary arteries open,
maintain your blood pressure within normal limits, and
lower abnormal cholesterol and other blood fats.

As important as any or all of the above is our new
knowledge about heart function and our appreciation of
the importance of lifestyle in preventing not only a first

heart attack, but also a recurrence. All the preventive measures described above are now more important than ever.

If you've survived one heart attack, you must seriously and with dedication do everything you can to prevent a second one. You may not be as lucky next time around. Remember, coronary bypass surgery, angioplasties, or any of the new "miracle" interventions are not cures. They're simply holding measures to buy enough time for you to reduce your risk factors to prevent or delay being stricken again. You're being given a second chance. Take it.

What to Remember about Heart Attacks

1. Heart attacks are the number-one killer in most of the developed world.
2. Although the exact cause is not known, controlling the known risk factors is protective.
3. The most important risk factors are abnormal cholesterol and other blood fats, untreated hypertension, use of tobacco, obesity, diabetes, a bad family history of premature heart disease, physical inactivity, high homocysteine levels, and certain infections.
4. Persons without any of these risk factors are not necessarily immune from heart disease.
5. Chest symptoms on exertion (angina pectoris) usually precede a heart attack by days, weeks, months, or years.

6. Many heart attacks cause sudden death, but vulnerable persons can be identified by specific heart tests.

7. A normal ECG does not exclude the presence of heart disease. A stress test is often required to make the diagnosis.

8. There are now several procedures that can successfully restore blood flow to the heart before and during a heart attack.

9. The right lifestyle remains the cornerstone of prevention.

7

IMPOTENCE – THE NOT SO SILENT (ANYMORE) EPIDEMIC

Age, Hormones, or Performance Anxiety?

A ninety-year-old man with a healthy sex drive complained to his doctor that his passion for lovemaking was driving him crazy. The surprised physician asked, "And you're complaining?" "Yes. Please, I beg you. Do something about it!" As thoughts of saltpeter and other sexual suppressants flashed through the doctor's mind, his patient added, "You've got to move it down from my head to where it can do me some good."

Since the term *impotence* conveys the stigma of loss of manhood, doctors now often refer to it as "erectile dysfunction." But a rose by any other name . . .

Every man has his own definition of impotence. For some, it simply can't happen to them, no matter how obvious the symptoms: "Impotent? Me? You've got to be kidding. I'm as good as I ever was. Of course, right now I happen to have other things on my mind. I'm stressed out. All I need is a vacation." At the other end of the spectrum is the man who believes he's impotent because he can't always "get it up" on demand. Unless his performance is 100 percent, like it was when he was eighteen, he's convinced that he's got a problem. The worry feeds on itself, and sex ultimately becomes more of a challenge than a pleasure.

Impotence is not the same as a lack of desire, or premature ejaculation (when you "explode" or fizzle out as soon as you're put to the test). You're impotent when you're sexually aroused but your penis doesn't respond predictably.

An estimated 30 million men in this country are impotent, yet only 4 million seek treatment for it each year (that number is probably higher now that Viagra is available). I'm not sure how accurate these numbers are, since impotence is not the kind of thing men brag about, share with their closest friends, or even complain about to their doctor very often. Indeed, a spouse or partner is more apt to report her mate's impotence than he is. Unfortunately, she's not always reliable. The last time a woman asked me to do something about her husband's problem, he later confided to me that he had no trouble whatsoever making love to his girlfriend!

Impotence is by no means solely a consequence of aging. Although sexual prowess does decrease with age (about 5 percent of men are impotent at age forty, and one in four go limp by the time they reach sixty-five), the problem can and does occur early in life as well.

How Does an Erection Happen?

For a penis to become erect *on demand* (that's the sine qua non of normal sexual function) and stay that way long enough to consummate the act, a host of physical and emotional factors must be intact.

- You must be free of serious sexual hang-ups that turn you off or prevent you from being turned on.
- Your body must be making enough male hormone, testosterone, for you to respond to a thought, a sexy sight, or the stimulation of an erotic zone. When your testosterone level is too low, the most passionate advance from the sexiest woman won't do a thing either to your brain or your penis. (That's why harems hire eunuchs.)
- Designated areas of the brain must be free of disease to be able to interpret your sexual desire and send the appropriate message down to where it counts.
- These signals travel along pathways in the spinal column and end up in the penis. The nerves that carry them must be intact, and the route they follow must be free of obstruction.
- When the "Hey, let's go" impulses reach the genital area, they relax muscles within the penis, permitting blood to flow into the corpora cavernosa in the penis, two spongy chambers that run throughout its length. The corpora are made up of smooth muscle, supporting fibrous tissue, veins, arteries, and lots of empty space. When they fill with blood, the penis becomes

stiff. But for that to happen, not only must the muscles relax, but the arteries that carry the blood to the penis must also be free of obstructing plaques.

So sexual potency involves a complicated chain of events. A break in any link, whether due to psychological, vascular, or neurological causes, can lead to impotence.

What Causes Impotence?

• **Age:** To what extent does age, independent of other risk factors, contribute to impotence? Although testosterone production diminishes as a man gets older, that's where the analogy with menopause ends. Estrogen output drops dramatically when menses ends, but testosterone levels in aging men are usually high enough to maintain some libido and erectile function. Unless there is some other cause for their impotence (see below), men in their eighties and older can continue to produce sperm and remain potent. However, the amount and the force of the ejaculate are diminished (but few elderly men care about that). Too many men, dissatisfied with their sexual performance, resort to testosterone supplements by shot, cream, patch, or orally. Such measures are usually not necessary, and the extra testosterone can, at least theoretically, activate a dormant prostate cancer.

• **Psychological factors:** There is some physical basis for impotence in 80 percent of cases; the problem is basically psychological in the remaining 20 percent. If an erotic dream provokes one or more erections during the night, with or without an orgasm, but you can't perform with a sexual partner, your impotence is probably psychological. However, older men who are impotent for physical reasons may experience a spontaneous erection early in the morning when their bladder is full. When an impotent man puts this unexpected bonus to the test, he usually finds that the erection fades as mysteriously as it came, without ever fulfilling its promise. Leonardo da Vinci described it this way: "The penis has a mind of its own. Often the man is asleep, and it is awake, and many times the man is awake and it is asleep."

There's yet another diagnostic criterion. If you can't get it up or keep it up with any partner whom you find sexy, but you do very well when alone and masturbating to the tune of some sexual fantasy, your problem is in your head. You've been aroused, the penis has received the message, the blood has flowed in, and the organ is erect. The reason it doesn't happen with a partner is obviously emotional. Don't waste your time and money on fancy vascular and neurological tests. See a psychologist. However, if your penis is never more than semi-erect during masturbation, and there are no emotional hang-ups, there is probably some underlying physical cause.

Many complex psychological and emotional factors can lead to impotence; few if any are due to the aging process per se. These hang-ups include parental, religious, or peer conditioning early in life that imbues sexual activity with guilt, frustration, embarrassment; stress;

the inability to deal with an intimate interpersonal relationship or to make a commitment; and anxiety about the consequences of sex (fear of a sexually transmitted disease or the belief that one's heart will not be able to withstand the stress). A relationship gone sour, the death of a spouse, panic at the prospect of performance failure, depression, and a host of other emotional states can also result in impotence. However, before you conclude that your erectile dysfunction is psychological, be sure to exclude all of the other causes described below.

• **Medication:** Sex and most drugs don't mix. Medications account for at least 25 percent of all cases of impotence. If your sexual performance leaves something to be desired, review every drug you're taking, whether it's a prescription item or one you've picked up over-the-counter. For example, beta-blockers, used to lower blood pressure, control palpitations, and treat various heart conditions (Inderal is the prototype), can cause impotence and a decreased libido. So can a variety of high-blood-pressure drugs. Even the antihistamine you're taking for your allergy can do it. Naproxen (Naprosyn), my favorite nonsteroidal anti-inflammatory agent that relieves all kinds of aches and pains, has also occasionally been implicated. In a minority of people, a slew of antidepressants and tranquilizers can interfere with normal brain metabolism and result in impotence. Phenylpropanolamine, the ingredient in some appetite suppressants and cold remedies, may decongest your penis as well as your nose. Even cimetidine (Tagamet), a very popular and effective anti-ulcer drug, can sometimes diminish desire, arousal, and orgasm—even in women. If you're diabetic, the vascular and neurological complications of the disease can prevent an erection, and so can the pill you're taking to lower your sugar. Men with prostate cancer become impotent when they're treated with female hormones, such as estrogen, as well as with the newer, effective antitestosterone agents.

• **Vascular disease:** As I indicated earlier, the sine qua non of an erection is adequate blood flow into the penis. Constantinus Africanus, a Latin scholar and doctor, summed it up 1,000 years ago with this observation: "When appetite arises, the heart generates a spirit that descends through the arteries, fills the hollow of the penis, and makes it hard and stiff." That "spirit" is blood! When the arteries feeding the penis are sufficiently narrowed or obstructed enough to reduce its crucial blood supply, the best efforts of the mind, the brain, the hormones, and the nerves will not produce an erection.

The most common vascular disorder resulting in impotence is arteriosclerosis (hardening of the arteries). Plaques in the arteries to the penis (and every other organ in the body) are the price you pay for a lifetime of eating a fat-rich diet, of untreated high blood pressure, of smoking, and of poorly controlled diabetes. If you have any one of these risk factors, you're four times more likely to become impotent. A high cholesterol level, especially an elevated LDL ("bad" cholesterol) and a low HDL ("good" cholesterol), are important predictors of impotence down the road. Statistically speaking, they are probably more significant than your testosterone level.

Blood supply to the penis can be reduced by physical injury to its arteries as well as by disease. It's estimated that 600,000 men in this country have been rendered impotent by trauma to their genitalia, sustained either at work or at play. The most vulnerable arteries are those that are damaged as they pass unprotected through the perineum (the area between the legs from the base of the scrotum to the anus) on their way to the penis. They can be affected in a number of ways. According to Dr. Irwin Goldstein, a noted authority on impotence, 100,000 men are impotent because the seat of their bicycle or the top tube of its frame damaged their penis. "Fifty percent of the penis is inside the body and attached to the bone that rests against the bicycle seat," Dr. Goldstein explains. "When you sit, you're putting your entire weight on the artery that supplies the penis. Let's say you're traveling at 7.5 miles an hour. That translates to a quarter-ton of weight crushing down on your penis." I must say that in all my years of bicycle riding, I never appreciated how much I was endangering my marital bliss. If you're a bike rider and are having potency problems, consider horseback riding instead.

Decreased blood flow into the penis is not the only vascular cause of impotence. During sex, what goes in must eventually come out. The surge of blood that makes the penis erect must obviously leave at some point—the later the better. This exit takes place through the veins in the penis. However, when the veins remove the blood too quickly (usually because they are dilated like varicose veins in the legs), they create what is called a venous leak—and impotence.

- **Nerve disorders:** You need an intact nervous system to have successful erections. The messages that nerve fibers carry from the brain cause the penile smooth muscles to relax, allowing blood to flow into it. Anything that hurts these nerves can prevent those vital signals from reaching their destination. Injury to the spinal cord or pelvis can damage them, they may be cut during prostate surgery (the newer nerve-sparing operations cause such injury much less often), or they can be destroyed by local radiation (especially in the treatment of prostate cancer and other tumors in the pelvis or genitourinary tract).

- **Diabetes:** Almost 50 percent of diabetic males have erectile dysfunction. Poor control of sugar levels over the years leads not only to arterial blockages that cut down the flow of blood into the penis, but also to nerve damage (diabetic neuropathy) that makes erection difficult or impossible.

- **Other causes:** Virtually any chronic disease can leave you impotent. Some of the more common illnesses associated with impotence are multiple sclerosis (because it affects the nerves), strokes (when vital areas of the brain are injured), kidney disease (especially in patients with renal failure undergoing dialysis), chronic alcoholism, and cigarette smoking. (One study reported a 56 percent incidence of impotence in smokers as compared to 21 percent in nonsmokers.)

Evaluating Impotence

Times have changed. Impotence is no longer permanent. Afflicted men now have many treatment options, and more are on the way. But therapy must be tailored to the individual. It can't be shotgun, like "Here's a pill" or "Take this injection," regardless of what's causing the impotence. Every man with this problem should be asked to provide a detailed personal and medical history and should undergo a thorough physical exam. (It's a good idea for your spouse or sexual partner to come along, at least for the history-taking portion.) If some medication is the culprit, stop it and you're cured. Sometimes a simple observation during the physical can lead to an immediate diagnosis. For example, inspecting the penis may reveal Peyronie's disease, with which one prominent American is said to be affected. This is a curvature of the penis caused by scar tissue. Although it usually only affects the angle of penetration or causes painful erections, it is sometimes responsible for impotence. The physical exam may uncover diabetes, or a vascular or neurological problem. Blood tests, in addition to identifying sugar and hormone levels, also reveal whether or not the blood fats are normal. (When the level of testosterone is measured, the blood should be drawn in the morning.) High cholesterol, low HDL, and/or high LDL may point to the reason for an existing vascular problem.

Doctors used to monitor nocturnal erections because they believed that if you have an erection under any circumstances, even an involuntary one, you're fine physically and the impotence is psychological. That's not always true, so I no longer recommend this procedure. I prefer an ultrasound test of the penis done by a good urologist. It's noninvasive and provides important information about penile structure and blood supply.

Treating Impotence

The treatment of impotence depends on its cause. If the culprit is a drug or medication, discontinue it, change it, or alter the dosage, if possible. If the testosterone level is low, hormonal supplements may solve the problem. If there is vascular disease, arterial obstructions can often be relieved surgically and venous leaks repaired. Quitting smoking cigarettes and cutting out the booze may help if the nerves and arteries have not been irreversibly damaged. When psychological factors are contributing to impotence (this diagnosis is essentially one of exclusion, after all other causes have been ruled out), counseling and treatment can help. You can benefit from such guidance even when there is a physical component to the problem.

Always opt for the least invasive therapy first. It's obviously better to take a pill than to have a surgical implant. The therapeutic scene is rapidly changing. Sildenafil (Viagra) is the "hottest" recent approach to the treatment of impotence. It had a very impressive track record in prerelease trials both in this country and in Europe, with an 80 percent success rate even among diabetics. I have never been so overwhelmed by phone calls after the introduction of a new drug in all my years of practice as I was with Viagra. As soon as the news broke that it was available by prescription, I received as many as fifteen calls a day—from the most unexpected sources. Men who had never before intimated that they'd had any performance problem called for an "emergency" prescription of the drug—so did their wives, and even their girlfriends. Women called to ask whether Viagra would enhance their libido so that they could keep up with their reinvigorated husbands. (There is some evidence that it may.) I said earlier in this section that most men don't complain about impotence, or do anything about it. But Viagra has changed all that. There is no longer the same shyness and secrecy about the problem now that you can buy a magic pill to cure it!

Millions of Viagra pills are being sold in this country and their success rate is somewhere between 60 and 70 percent. However, don't expect much from Viagra if the other forms of treatment for impotence, such as implants or penile injection, have failed.

Here is how Viagra works. Sexual arousal is normally accompanied by an increased concentration of a chemical called cyclic GMP in the penis. There is also an enzyme that breaks down this chemical. Viagra blocks the action of that enzyme, leaving plenty of the cyclic GMP in the penis to ensure an erection. It also relaxes the muscles that control the entry of blood into the penis. Although the manufacturer claims that Viagra works in about an hour, many of my patients have told me that it may take as long as two hours to work, and some have found the window of opportunity to remain open for as long as six hours. One of Viagra's advantages is that it won't do much unless you're aroused. So if you're told "No, dear, not tonight" and have already taken the pill, you won't have to endure an unwanted erection. Viagra should be taken on an empty stomach, and it has only occasional minor, temporary side effects such as blurred vision (but then, you won't be reading when it's working, will you?), headache, flushing, the inability to distinguish between the colors blue and green, mild headache (now it's you, not your spouse, who'll complain about it), and dyspepsia.

Viagra tablets come in 25-, 50-, and 100-milligram strength, and it's expensive. Some insurance plans will pay for it, others won't. I usually prescribe the 50-milligram dose to start, but I have found that most men need 100 milligrams. There are a few caveats, however. Take the lower strength while you're on erythromycin or an antifungal agent such as ketoconazole or itraconazole. Like Viagra, these medications are metabolized through the liver enzyme system. Also—and this is very important—don't take Viagra if you are using any nitrate drug for angina pectoris. The combination of Viagra and one of these coronary dilator drugs can drop your blood pressure to dangerously low levels. There have been several deaths, heart attacks, and strokes in men after using Viagra. These have not been due to a direct action of the medication itself. Those needing the pill are older men, many of whom have cardiac, neurological, and vascular problems, and may therefore be unable to withstand the sudden stress of sexual activity to which they are no longer accustomed. Also, some may have been taking the forbidden nitrates along with theViagra.

Don't give up on Viagra if it doesn't work on your first try. Try it four or five times.

Although Viagra has turned out to be the most widely used urological drug ever, its long-term consequences remain to be determined. Perhaps the most fascinating aspect of the Viagra story is its serendipitous discovery. The Pfizer scientists who developed it were actually looking for a new pill to improve angina pectoris. They found that Viagra didn't do much for chest pain, but the test subjects, at least the men among them, loved it and held on to the unused supplies when the study was finished! And no wonder, after what it so unexpectedly did for them! (Darn it—why didn't I buy Pfizer stock back then?)

Topical nitroglycerin: If Viagra doesn't work, there is another option. As a cardiologist, I often have occasion to prescribe nitroglycerin for patients with coronary artery disease. A small tablet dissolved under the tongue relieves the chest pain (angina pectoris) by dilating the arteries in the heart. Some patients have told me, and there have been confirming reports in the medical literature, that when they rub nitroglycerin cream or ointment on their penis, its vessels dilate and produce an erection. However, since this drug also widens blood vessels in the head, one of its side effects is a transient headache. So it's possible that both you and your partner may develop headaches from the nitroglycerin!

Vacuum pumps: The first option I recommend if Viagra or other medications aren't effective is the vacuum device. It's effective for virtually every type of impotence in which there is enough blood available. These devices, the best known of which is the Osbon, consist of an acrylic cylinder that's placed over the flaccid penis and attached to a pump that draws air out of the cylinder. This creates a vacuum that sucks blood into the penis, and two or three elastic rings placed snugly on the base of the penis keep it there. You need to squeeze the pump handle only a few times to create enough of a vacuum. Once an erection has occurred, the penis is removed from the cylinder. It now stands proudly on its own, albeit cool, slightly purple, and with somewhat less sensation than normal. The erection persists even after the orgasm, because the blood is still locked into the penis by the elastic bands at its base. When these are removed, blood and the ejaculate leave the penis, and the erection subsides.

There are several drawbacks to the vacuum device. First of all, it's not terribly romantic. Although one soon becomes adept at its use, it means interrupting foreplay and concentrating on a mechanical maneuver. Still, it does make intercourse possible, and most couples adjust to the inconvenience. Another disadvantage, for those who want to make babies, is that the ejaculate is trapped within the penis, along with the blood, until the rings are removed. At that point, however, the organ is too flaccid to permit penetration, so the sperm is wasted. Don't leave the rings on your turgid organ for longer than thirty minutes. Interfering with the blood supply for a longer period of time can be harmful. A vacuum pump costs $300 to $400. It's worth trying. I understand that the manufacturer will refund your money if it doesn't work.

Penile injections: Several injectable drugs are now available to promote erections. All of them work by relaxing the smooth muscle in the penis so that blood can enter and make it erect. The doctor first gives you a small test dose of whichever drug (or combinations) he or she plans to use. The quality and duration of the resulting erection are then noted. If they're satisfactory, you will be taught how to inject the medication into the body of the penis. The technique is usually no more painful than a pinprick, and most patients have no problem learning how to do it. There are several drawbacks to penile injections: the need to inject yourself; the manual dexterity or adequate vision necessary to do it (not every older man can fill a syringe correctly and then inject himself); since these drugs are vascular dilators, they can cause a temporary drop in blood pressure, which may not be well tolerated by the elderly or those taking other blood pressure–lowering agents; repeated injections into the body of the penis can cause scarring, so don't take them if you already have Peyronie's disease (a condition in which the penis is curved); if you're taking anticoagulants (blood thinners) you may bleed after the injection; and priapism, a painful erection, may occur, which persists for hours.

"Priapism" comes from the legend of Priapus, the son

of Aphrodite and Dionysus of Greek mythology. Statues erected (no pun intended) in his honor endow him very well indeed. An erection that continues for too long can reduce the blood supply to the penis or cause clots to form within it and permanently injure it. It's too much of a good thing. Papaverine is the drug most likely to cause priapism (although cases have also been reported with Viagra). Before you leave your doctor's office, full of enthusiasm, syringe in hand, all set to inject yourself and enjoy an erection, ask for some 5 milligram tablets of terbutaline. If the injection works but your erection refuses to quit after two hours, take one of these tablets every fifteen minutes (but no more than three of them) to get rid of the priapism. This will work in 20 to 30 percent of cases. If the erections persists for four hours, go back to your doctor. He'll irrigate your stubborn organ with a solution of salt water and phenylephrine.

Although you can excuse yourself when foreplay has had the desired effect, retire to the bathroom, and inject yourself surreptitiously in anticipation of sexual pleasure, this technique, like the vacuum pump, also interferes with spontaneity. It has the advantage over Viagra in working almost immediately.

Satisfaction with and adherence to injection therapy is about the same as with the vacuum device—men prefer one or the other, but a substantial number are soon fed up with both and stop using them. Unlike the case with Viagra, you needn't be sexually aroused for either the vacuum pump or the injections to be effective.

Urethral medication: Unlike the papaverine, phentolamine, and prostaglandin E1 injections into the body of the penis, you can put some alprostadil gel or a small pellet into the urethra (at the tip of the penis) using a plastic applicator. You'll see a response within thirty minutes. According to one study of 1,500 men who used this technique (marketed as MUSE), two-thirds achieved a number-four erection, that is, sufficient for intercourse, or, if they were really lucky, a number 5, a really rigid one. Other assessments of alprostadil have not been so impressive. Italian researchers found that increased volume of blood into the penis did not always result in hardness, just a larger size. When they applied their "penile stress test" (a one-kilogram weight is dangled from the penis) to the subjects receiving MUSE, they found that the organ buckled in more than 100 of the 123 men tested. In other words, "Complete rigidity was not achieved."

If you try the MUSE system, be prepared for the cost. MUSE sex doesn't come cheap. Each session will set you back between $30 and $40. Frankly, some patients have told me that this tablet hurts them more than the injections described above. Few men in my own practice still use MUSE.

Penile implants and other surgery: There are some circumstances where no medication will work and a physical approach is required. For example, a drug that relaxes the smooth muscle to allow blood into your penis won't do much good if your arteries are obstructed. Or if the interior of the penis itself has been so scarred by infection that it can't accommodate the necessary volume of blood, no medication will help, either. In these circumstances, you still have the popular surgical option.

There are three different kinds of operations for impotence. The surgeon can insert a device or implant into the penis that will make it erect, he or she can reconstruct damaged arteries within the penis, or the varicose veins within the penis that are responsible for the "venous leak," the rapid exit of the blood from that organ, can be repaired.

Two-thirds of the implants used today are inflatable and collapsible—blown up on demand. They are also paired, and are filled with fluid before sex is to begin. The implants are connected by tubes to a fluid-filed reservoir and small pump, which is surgically inserted under the skin in the scrotum. When the pump is discreetly squeezed, the flaccid penis stands up. The main advantage of the inflatable implants over the rigid ones is that they do not leave the penis in a state of perpetual erection. These operations used to cost upward of $20,000; they are now done for under $2,000.

Implants may also consist of a pair of flexible rods inserted into the corpora cavernosa, the parallel hollow chambers that run the length of the penis. They don't make the penis any wider or longer; they just keep it firm enough to penetrate. Their insertion results in a constant state of erection. That's not as much fun as you think. The penis never goes down, forcing the recipient to reposition it from the downward direction to the upright. When you wear a bathing suit at the beach, people may think you're showing off.

There are problems with these operations even in the best of hands. Infection is not uncommon; prostheses sometimes break down and need to be removed, and that means another operation.

When impotence is due to a "venous leak," tying off the varicose veins in the penis sometimes cures the problem, but this procedure is not very popular among urologists.

Other currently available medical therapy: Over the years, several medications and herbs have been touted for the treatment of impotence, ranging from Spanish fly to ginseng. I have been unable to find documentation that any of them work. For a while, yohimbine was in vogue, but recent reports conclude that it is ineffective. I suggest you avoid it because of its adverse side effects, mainly a rise or fall in blood pressure. Dopamine, some of the selective serotonin reuptake inhibitors (SSRIs) such as Prozac, and trazodone, a tranquilizer, have also been said to be effective, but these claims have not been confirmed by scientific studies. There was one interesting report in which thirty-one impotent men volunteered to try aromatherapy for their problem. There was a measurable response when they sniffed lavender (with or without added cola and oriental spice). Older men preferred a vanilla scent. Try it. You've got nothing to lose.

Promising treatments on the horizon: Two new drugs are expected to be approved in this country in the near future. They work in different ways, and have had varying rates of success in early trials. However, they both require an adequate blood flow into the penis in order to be effective.

Apomorphine (to be marketed as Spontane in the United States) produces the best results in men with psychogenic impotence. It acts directly on the area of the brain that triggers erections, and has been found to be 70 percent effective in recent trials. A vivid imagination is not enough to activate this drug; you need to be physically stimulated in order for it to work. The problem with apomorphine is that, aside from turning erotic thoughts into penile reality, it also causes nausea and vomiting. So the manufacturer, the Tap Company, developed an apomorphine preparation that dissolves under the tongue. It's absorbed so slowly that it does away with impotence yet is free of the undesirable side effects of the oral form.

Another area of promising research is the conversion of phentolamine, one of the drugs now available only by injection, into an oral preparation (to be marketed in the United States as Vasomax). It also requires erotic stimulation, and takes from twenty to forty minutes to work. Vasomax will probably be marketed before the year 2000. Its effectiveness, however, is not expected to exceed 40 percent.

Finally, here's something Rube Goldberg might have come up with. Italian doctors have developed a penile pacemaker that's currently being evaluated. It consists of a tiny box containing a battery-operated microchip that's inserted into the scrotum and connected to sensors at the base of the penis. When a man is sexually stimulated, the chip activates the nerves that relax the smooth muscle of the penis, allowing blood to fill it and produce an erection. The operation takes about two hours; it costs about the same as a heart pacemaker ($7,000 to $10,000), and the batteries last for years.

What to Remember about Impotence

1. Some 30 million men in the United States suffer from impotence. Most of them are older and their problem stems from several different diseases. Aging is *not* a disease, and impotence is not its inevitable consequence.
2. The causes of impotence are primarily psychological in only 20 percent of cases. The majority are due to medications, trauma to the genital area, vascular problems, and neurological disorders.
3. Most cases of impotence can be successfully treated, either by drugs or devices. The latest breakthrough is sildenafil (Viagra), which is taken orally. Millions of tablets have already been taken in this country. Though generally safe and effective, it must not be taken with coronary dilator drugs such as short- and long-acting nitrates. Alternatives to Viagra are the vacuum pump, various methods of delivering drugs directly into the penis, surgical implants, and corrective surgery for vascular problems in the penis.
4. Testosterone deficiency is not a major cause of impotence. Most men continue to make enough testosterone to keep them potent and able to produce

sperm until they are well into their eighties. The widespread use of testosterone supplements is usually unnecessary, and not without danger.

5. Several newer oral agents are on the horizon and are expected to be available within the next year or two.

8

INSOMNIA

News You Can Use
to Help You Snooze

My mother never slept. She used to remind me of that, without fail, every single morning of my life. "I didn't sleep a wink last night, not a wink," accompanied my orange juice at breakfast. My mother was not a complainer; she was simply stating the fact that she hadn't slept. Throughout my childhood, she never, ever did. But strangely enough, whenever I was sick, and came to her bedroom during the night, she was always asleep, or so it seemed to me. Her eyes were closed and she was snoring. But I guess I was wrong, because when I apologized for waking her (it took several nudges), she'd invariably say, "Don't be silly. You didn't wake me. I wasn't sleeping."

I never understood why my father, my brother, all my aunts and uncles, and I all slept at night, yet my poor mother didn't. I thought this might be an affliction of mothers, so I asked my friends whether their mothers slept. Most of them said yes, a few didn't know, and the rest thought that my question was kind of bizarre. So I concluded, while growing up, that although some people do sleep at night, many mothers do not.

You can imagine my surprise when as a medical student I learned that my mother was almost unique in the annals of medicine, for there was only one other family whose members also never slept. *The New England Journal of Medicine* reported that fourteen persons in a clan in Bologna, Italy, all died from chronic insomnia. The last survivor was a fifty-three-year-old man who passed away after not sleeping "a wink" for nine months. Impressive, but not to be compared with my mother, who never slept throughout her entire life of ninety-four years!

I now believe that although Mother may conceivably have had what is called idiopathic insomnia, a neurological disorder characterized by a lifetime of poor sleeping, she was more likely one of the 5 percent of people who, when studied at a sleep laboratory, fall asleep within twenty minutes, remain asleep for six to seven hours, and wake up complaining that they hadn't slept at all!

What Is Insomnia?

Insomnia does not refer to the number of hours you sleep. What counts is whether you wake up refreshed and able to function normally the next day. For example, my friend Dr. Michael DeBakey, the renowned heart surgeon, insists that he needs only four hours' sleep (shades of my mother!). On the other hand, if I have less than five hours, I'm tired, irritable, and unable to concentrate the next day. I have even been known to doze while talking on the telephone. You have insomnia, then, because you need more sleep than you're getting, whether it's four hours or ten, and/or because its quality, regardless of duration, is so poor that you feel wiped out the next day.

How We Sleep

Mammals vary considerably in their sleep patterns. For example, whales nod off while swimming, horses and elephants can sleep standing up, and some animals doze with their eyes wide open. (I swear that some of my students do too.)

Sleep is a dynamic process, more than a matter of merely closing your eyes and waiting for your body to slow down for a few hours. In humans, a night's sleep consists of four to six cycles, each of which is composed of two distinct and very different alternating states: non–rapid eye movement (non-REM), and rapid eye movement (REM), when the muscles controlling the eyes roll slowly or move in rapid bursts. There are four stages of non-REM sleep. As you go from one to four, the level of sleep becomes more restful, the muscles throughout your body relax, and your heart rate and blood pressure drop. While sleeping in stage one, a pin dropping can wake you up; in stage four, it may take several rolling pins to rouse you. After the fourth stage, the process is reversed, sleep becomes lighter and lighter and you move back to stage one. Before the return to stage one of the non-REM sleep, your body switches to the much lighter REM sleep for about five minutes. That's when you dream. You then start the second cycle, and continue alternating non-REM and REM sleep phases in each of the six cycles during the night. In the later cycles, the deep sleep stages (three and four) are shorter, and the REM or dreaming phases longer. That means you get your deepest sleep during the first third of the night, and most of your dreams later. How well you sleep, and whether or not you have insomnia, depend on the balance between the REM and non-REM components in each of these four to six sleep cycles.

The Consequences of Insomnia

Insomnia can be temporary, lasting only a few nights, as happens with jet lag or a change in your work schedule; it can persist for weeks, usually because of some illness; or it can be chronic, occurring most nights and continuing for a month or more.

Insomnia is usually manifested by:

- trouble falling asleep (taking a half hour or more to do so)
- awakening during the night and being unable to return to sleep
- awakening too early in the morning
- agitated and nonrefreshing sleep

Sleep and the Senior Citizen

In young adults, each sleep cycle lasts from sixty to ninety minutes. These become shorter as we grow older, and stages one and two of non-REM sleep, the lighter kind, last longer than the more profound stages three and four. Some older persons never slip into stage four. Remember that the more stages three and four of the non-REM sleep you get, the more rested you will be. (Dream time in REM sleep doesn't change with the years.) Because there is a longer time spent during which sleep is superficial, older persons awaken more frequently during the night, as often as 150 times or more, although they may remember only eight or ten such awakenings. They usually go back to sleep, but these interruptions, remembered or not, interfere with the quality of sleep and account for some of the consequences of insomnia. Young adults, by contrast, usually awaken only five or six times a night. If you add to these multiple, momentary awakenings, the need that most older men have to empty their bladders during the night, you see why so many elderly persons complain of "insomnia."

Besides these important biological changes, there are many other reasons why older persons have problems sleeping—to which retirement, bereavement, medications, chronic illness, and financial concerns all contribute.

The obvious results of insomnia are fatigue, irritability, and poor performance at work and play. But your resulting sleepiness can also affect those around you. The National Highway Traffic Safety Administration estimates that more than 200,000 car accidents every year are due to fatigue. Would you feel safe on a plane piloted by an insomniac or guided into the airport by a sleepy air-traffic controller? How would you enjoy being on a train or bus, or in a taxi, driven by my mother or anyone else who hadn't had a good night's sleep?

And there are other complications of insomnia. Memory, the ability to learn, to make logical decisions or mathematical calculations, are also impaired. There are economic consequences too. Insomnia is a significant contributor to absenteeism. People just don't feel up to working when they're worn out for lack of sleep. The immune system is also impaired by sleep deprivation, since sleep is considered to be an important factor in the body's ability to overcome infection and other disorders. Finally, people with chronic sleeping problems are much more likely to develop psychiatric difficulties.

Causes of Insomnia

There are many causes of insomnia at every age. These include:

• **Depression, stress, anxiety,** and other psychiatric disorders are probably the most important foilers of sleep at any age. With lots of problems, real or fancied, on your mind, you're apt to have trouble falling and staying asleep.

• **Female gender.** Women often find their sleep habits less satisfying, especially in relation to their menstrual cycle, during pregnancy, after giving birth, and at the onset of menopause.

• **Jet lag.** When your job calls for frequent travel across time zones, your body's sleep/wake schedule is chronically upset.

• **Changes in your environment** can interfere with a good night's sleep: noise from passing traffic, airplanes overhead, a neighbor's television next door, your bedroom being too hot, too cold, or too bright.

• **Sleep apnea** and other breathing disorders account for more than half the cases of insomnia and affect almost 20 million Americans. The word *apnea* is derived from the Greek meaning "want of breath." It's characterized by hundreds of interruptions of breathing during the night, of which you may be unaware. The diagnosis is usually made by a spouse or other bedmate who complains of the loud snoring, one of the hallmarks of sleep apnea. In addition to causing insomnia, sleep apnea increases the risk of heart attack and stroke due to the lack of oxygen to the heart and brain when breathing pauses.

• **Medical problems** that cause pain or discomfort can all interfere with a good night's sleep. The most common are cancer, arthritis, heart failure, emphysema, kidney disease, prostate problems, heartburn, hot flashes, Parkinson's disease, an overactive thyroid, the "restless legs" syndrome, and peptic ulcers.

- **Medications** can prevent you from falling asleep, or cause you to wake up too soon. Examples are stimulant drugs such as Ritalin or amphetamines, weight-reduction pills that contain ephedrine or pseudoephedrine, decongestants, thyroid supplements, bronchodilators for asthma, and alphamethyldopa (Aldomet)—a blood pressure pill (formerly more widely used than it is today).
- **Caffeine** taken with dinner, later in the evening, or at bedtime may interfere with sleep.
- **Alcohol** at bedtime may help you fall asleep, but it usually wakes you up later.
- **Cigarettes** are a common cause of insomnia (and virtually everything else that's bad for the body).
- **A long nap** in the afternoon or evening may make it more difficult to sleep during the night.

People over sixty are more apt to complain of insomnia than are younger persons. They have more trouble falling asleep, they awaken more often, and then find it harder to return to sleep.

Treating and Preventing Insomnia

It's one thing to know why older people don't sleep as well; it's quite another to do something about it. There is no easy solution because the aging process proceeds at a different pace in different people and affects each of us differently. If you're one of the 35 million Americans who has trouble sleeping, remember that age is not the only culprit. Look for and eliminate or control as many of the other possible contributing factors listed above as you can. Here are some general measures to help you sleep, no matter how old or how young you are:

• **Exercise regularly,** preferably aerobically, for twenty to thirty minutes *in the late afternoon,* but not during the four to six hours before bedtime, and never just before you go to sleep. You sleep better when your body temperature is low, and exercise raises it. Body temperature normally rises during the day and falls at night, but in someone with insomnia, there is less of a temperature spread; they're not as warm in the daytime or as cool at night. If you warm your body with a workout in the late afternoon, it will cool down when you're ready for sleep.

• **Don't become preoccupied** with sleeping, and don't work at trying to fall asleep. That will only keep you awake.

• **Psychotherapy** and the appropriate antidepressants can help insomnia.

• **A good massage** will do as much for you as any other intervention, physical or chemical. Teach your husband (wife, girlfriend, or boyfriend) how to do it.

• **Sex** relaxes some people and helps them sleep; it stimulates or worries others and keeps them awake. Decide whether you're an A.M. or a P.M. type and act accordingly.

• **Rotate your work shifts** in a forward sequence: first work days, then evenings, and then nights. Remain on each shift for at least three weeks. Switching more often than that doesn't allow your biological clock to adjust.

- **Older people tend to be more sensitive to caffeine,** but anyone with a sleeping problem should avoid it late in the day. That means no coffee, sodas, chocolate, tea (except chamomile, which can help you sleep), or diet pills. I advise my patients not to have more than three cups of coffee a day and never later than lunchtime. Even if you have no trouble sleeping after drinking coffee at or near bedtime, chances are it wakens you more often and reduces the soundness or quality of your sleep.

- **Forget your nightcap.** Alcohol may help you nod off, but you won't sleep as soundly, and you are more likely to awaken during the night. Drink a glass of warm milk instead (the natural I-tryptophan it contains promotes sleep) and then have a warm bath for twenty minutes or so. (Note: If your prostate is large and you have to empty your bladder too often for comfort, don't drink any fluids for two hours before bedtime.)

- **Don't smoke before bedtime.** Nicotine is a stimulant; it raises blood pressure, makes the heart beat faster, and causes your brain to be more active.

- **You may satisfy your hunger pangs** with a light snack at bedtime, but avoid heavy, spicy, or high-fat foods. They increase gastric acidity and give you indigestion.

- **A proper diet** low in fat and with lots of salad, fruits, vegetables, whole grain, and fiber will contribute to good health and good sleep.

- **If you haven't slept well lately,** don't try to make up for it by napping during the next day. That will only aggravate your problem the following night.

- **Keep your bedroom a little cooler** than the rest of your home. You will sleep better when your body temperature drops a little. In the summertime, your bedroom should be air-cooled, if possible. It should also be dark. If it isn't, wear eyeshades.

- **Review with your doctor all the medications you're taking.** Either discontinue any that can contribute to your insomnia, or take them earlier in the day. I've listed earlier in this section some commonly used drugs that can interfere with sleep.

- **Remove any clocks that chime or click loudly** from your bedroom. If your favorite timepiece isn't noisy, you may keep it in the bedroom, but not where you can see it. You don't want to be reminded, as you toss and turn, how late it is. If you live near an airport or on a busy street, buy yourself some earplugs. Soundproof windows are expensive, and won't do much good if you open them for fresh air during the night.

- **Don't encourage friends** and business associates to call you late in the evening. The conversation may be troubling and/or stimulating enough to keep you awake.

- **Go to bed and wake up at approximately the same time every day whenever possible.** Your body likes a regular schedule, whether it's eating, moving your bowels, or sleeping. Don't sleep in on weekends, despite how tempting it is. Doing so can upset your body clock.

- **If your mattress is lumpy or your pillow uncomfortable, get new ones.** Make sure that your pajamas or nightgown are loose and comfortable. Some patients rave about the Dux mattress (it's very expensive), and the

Tempurpedic (more reasonably priced). The latter conforms to the shape of your body, and the manufacturer allows you to try it for a month or so. If it doesn't help your sleep, they will take it back and refund your money.

- **There are many different tapes** available to help you sleep. They play music, some other soothing sound such as ocean surf, a waterfall, or rain on a hot tin roof. There are also narrative tapes with hypnotic-like suggestion.

- **Don't go to bed before you're sleepy.** Wait it out somewhere other than your bedroom until you are.

- **Meditation is often helpful.** Dr. Herbert Benson's book *The Relaxation Response* can teach you how to do it. Also try counting your breaths (it's better than sheep). Patients have also been enthusiastic about the number-counting technique: close your eyes, relax your muscles, and count slowly down from 100 to 0, trying to visualize each number as you do so. Or you can try rhythmically contracting and relaxing various muscles at bedtime. If none of these measures work, ask your doctor to refer you to a facility where you can learn biofeedback and guided imagery—techniques that enable you to control your bodily functions.

- **Before resorting to sleeping pills,** ask your doctor to refer you to a sleep clinic where experts can identify and correct your specific sleep problems. For example, they may find out that you have sleep apnea. You should suspect this disorder if your spouse or bedmate complains of your snoring or says that your breathing is irregular and interspersed with long pauses. Sleep apnea can be corrected by a variety of techniques, ranging from simple flow of air into your nose in order to keep the air passages open to surgical removal of excess tissue in your throat that interferes with breathing.

What about Sleeping Pills?

In principle, I am opposed to sleeping pills. They can create problems of their own, especially in older people. Most of them are habituating and can leave you hooked. So try everything else before you ask for something to help you sleep. However, every now and then, a sleeping pill can tide you over some crisis. Be sure to get your doctor's approval before taking any medication, including herbs and over-the-counter remedies. This is especially important if you're pregnant or have any medical problems, especially of the kidneys or liver, or are troubled by sleep apnea.

I do not recommend over-the-counter medications, such as antihistamines. Although they may help you sleep, most of them leave you feeling like a zombie the next day. They also tend to give you a dry mouth. If your prostate is enlarged, they can cause urinary retention and send you to the emergency room to have your bladder emptied with a catheter. Some of these agents also worsen glaucoma, asthma, and other lung disorders, and most should not be taken with alcohol or with other sedatives and tranquilizers. Their only advantage is that you can get them without a prescription. The FDA has found the following brands to be safe and effective: Compoz, Nytol, Sleep-eze, Sominex, and Sominex-2. Three preparations with a different formulation, Unisom, Doxysom, and Ultra Sleep, are also effective. Still, I wouldn't take any of them for longer than two weeks without telling your doctor.

The sleep medications for which you need a doctor's prescription are classified in terms of how fast they work and how quickly they're eliminated from the body. If your main trouble is getting to sleep but you remain asleep once you do, you want something that works quickly—within the hour. Such a short-acting agent is preferable because it's eliminated promptly and doesn't accumulate in the body even if you take it for several nights. But a short-acting drug may not carry you through the night, especially if you tend to be an early morning riser. Any sleeping pill can produce what is called "rebound insomnia"—you have trouble getting to sleep after you stop taking it.

Below are some of the more widely prescribed sleeping preparations and their main characteristics. Don't take any of them for longer than three weeks. And never "borrow" one from anyone.

Triazolam, better known as *Halcion,* has acquired a bad reputation because of reports that it can cause short-term amnesia and violent behavior. None of my patients have ever developed these side effects, and I have found that Halcion works very well. However, I'm cautious about recommending it because of the litigious society in which we live.

The *benzodiazepine* family of drugs, of which Valium is the prototype, is perhaps the most widely prescribed for people with sleeping disorders. Don't drink alcohol if you're taking any of them regularly. *Flurazepam* is one of the oldest of these drugs. It's long-acting and may leave you drowsy the next day, but it's okay for anyone who also needs daytime sedation for any reason. *Temazepam* is good if you have trouble falling asleep but tend to wake up during the night and can't return to sleep. *Estazolam* is a popular, newer benzodiazepine. It gets you to sleep quickly and keeps you asleep without drowsiness the next day.

The newest agent on the market at the time of writing is *Ambien (zolpidem),* touted as non-habit forming, unlike all the others. It's still too early for me to say whether this is so, and whether Ambien is any better than the benzodiazepines.

Melatonin is the current rage for the treatment of insomnia in the elderly, especially among practitioners of alternative medicine. The rationale behind its use is that the brain makes less of this sleep-promoting hormone as we get older, and replacing it is the best way to treat insomnia. They may be right, but I am not aware of any scientific proof that melatonin is safe and effective when taken for any length of time. Although I have found it useful in helping me overcome jet lag, I do not recommend it on an ongoing basis.

DHEA, the "anti-aging" hormone, is very popular with some doctors, but not with me. DHEA, as Saddam Hussein might put it, is the "mother of all hormones." Made in the adrenal gland, it is the precursor of both estrogen and testosterone. Here's the theory behind its use: As we grow older, the body makes less and less DHEA. By the time you're eighty, you have only a fraction of the DHEA that was present when you were twenty. DHEA proponents argue that since there is less DHEA around as we age and we don't sleep as well, then poor sleep must be due to DHEA deficiency—so let's replace it. Logical perhaps, but simplistic. As is the case with melatonin, I'm not aware of any scientific studies proving that DHEA has an impact on insomnia at any age. I am also worried about its long-range effects. Given the suspected link between estrogen and breast cancer and the possibility that extra testosterone accelerates or even possibly causes prostate cancer, I am nervous about adding this hormone to anyone's regimen to help insomnia.

According to recent reports from Beijing, *acupuncture* improves sleep patterns. These observations have not been confirmed in this country, although an NIH panel has concluded that acupuncture can relieve certain levels of pain, notably pain that follows operations and dental procedures. However, if you suffer from insomnia, there's no downside to trying acupuncture, especially if you're on the verge of taking medication because everything else has failed.

Practitioners of Chinese medicine also suggest soaking your feet in warm water for twenty minutes at bedtime, and if that doesn't make you sleepy, have someone massage your feet with oil. Sounds good, but don't expect your insurance carrier to reimburse you for the oil.

What to Remember about Insomnia

1. Insomnia is a sleep pattern that leaves you tired the next day, regardless of how many hours you appear to have slept.

2. There are many causes of insomnia, including depression, medications, lifestyle, and other disease states.

3. Older people need as much sleep as they ever did, but they're less apt to get as good a night's sleep as they did when they were younger. That's because of changes in the nature of their biological sleep cycle.

4. Over-the-counter drugs are effective for mild insomnia, but the antihistamines among them leave you drowsy the next day and can cause other problems.

5. Hypnotics (i.e., sleeping pills) prescribed by your doctor should not be taken for more than two or three weeks. They are a crutch on which you can become dependent, and they never solve the underlying problem. Their long-term use can have a variety of harmful effects, especially in the elderly.

6. Melatonin and DHEA are currently being widely touted for the treatment of insomnia, but their efficiency has not been proved and the consequences of their prolonged use remain uncertain.

7. My mother never slept.

9

LIBIDO IN LIMBO

"No, dear, not tonight.
I have a headache."

Libido, the sex drive, is a very complex phenomenon determined by the interaction of many different factors—psychological, physical, hormonal, romantic, and environmental—at any age. Appetite for sex varies as widely as it does for food or alcohol. Just as some people can't wait for the next meal and others need to be reminded of it; or a drink before dinner is a must for some and entirely optional for others; so are there men and women whose sexual desires are never really satiated for very long, as well as those who can take it or leave it. Everyone's "sexostat" is set at a different level. (Don't bother looking up "sexostat" in the dictionary. You won't find it. I made it up.) However, unlike your innate metabolism, the sexostat can move up or down, depending largely on how and when you are aroused and what opportunities for sex present themselves.

The older you get, the less frequently you're apt to want or engage in sex. That decline is due to a subtle combination of diminished ardor (libido) and capability (potency), but it is not nearly as great as most younger people think. (Yes, Virginia, there is sex after sixty.) Libido and potency are not the same thing. Don't confuse waning desire with impotence. When you're impotent, you want to but can't; when you have no libido, you can but don't want to.

Why Your Libido May Be in Limbo

- You worry that having sex will give you a sexually transmitted disease, or that you will become pregnant, or that you will die because your bad heart can't take it.
- You grew up believing that sex is dirty or wrong.
- You feel guilty because you're cheating on your spouse or are in a relationship that is otherwise in conflict with your religious beliefs.
- You're taking some drug that suppresses libido, such as a blood pressure–lowering agent or a tranquilizer.
- You're worried that you won't perform satisfactorily—or at all.
- You're a chronic alcoholic or substance abuser.
- You don't think about sex much because you really have no opportunity to engage in it.

- Your spouse or partner is either impotent or disinterested, and so your own flames aren't fanned.
- You're depressed, worried, fatigued, or preoccupied with other problems.
- You're weak, or in pain, or concerned about some other disease from which you are suffering.

These are just a few of the causes of reduced desire for physical love. Normal libido does decrease as we get older, but it's usually gradual and subtle. The degree and pace varies from person to person. I have known men and women in their sixties who progressively and imperceptibly became more interested in golf than in sex; and others, much older, whose passion remained undiminished. I remember one eighty-four-year-old man who asked for an emergency appointment because he had been unable to have an erection the night before and was worried that he was becoming impotent.

What to Do about a Decreased Libido

Eighty-nine percent of couples in their sixties and 80 percent in their seventies remain sexually interested and active to some extent. And despite the drop in their level of female hormones, more than half of women have the same or greater degree of sexual activity after menopause.

That leaves almost 50 percent of women with lowered libido once their periods end. If you're one of them, you should be on estrogen replacement therapy (ERT) unless there's some contraindication. But be sure to take progesterone along with it in order to reduce the risk of cancer of the uterus (unless you've had a hysterectomy, in which case you don't need it). Estrogen replacement will make you feel better; it will improve the quality and enjoyment of sex by reducing vaginal dryness that makes penetration painful. This "moisturizing" decreases the chances of vaginal infection, and speeds up clitoral reaction time as well as the frequency with which the uterus contracts during an orgasm, thus increasing your pleasure.

Despite all these positive effects, estrogen may not increase libido per se because (and this may surprise you) *estrogen deficiency is not the major factor in loss of desire at this time of life*. Lack of sex drive is mainly due to abnormally low levels of *testosterone* (male hormone). Testosterone lack in a woman? Am I serious? Yes. Here's why:

Throughout life, both sexes make some of the other's hormones. Thankfully, women make mostly estrogen and just a little testosterone, while men produce lots of testosterone and only a touch of estrogen. But those small quantities make a big difference. Testosterone is largely responsible for the sex drive in men *and* women. After menopause, the relatively tiny amount of testosterone normally produced by females does not usually decrease, but it can—by as much as two-thirds. When it does, a woman's sex drive is impaired or lost. A combination of estrogen/progesterone and testosterone will help restore libido, increase energy, and improve mood.

The most commonly prescribed pills with this formulation are Estratest, and Premarin with methyl testosterone.

Progesterone alone, by contrast, decreases libido even in premenopausal women by interfering with the production of testosterone. That's why older contraceptives that contained progesterone dampened libido. If your sex urge is lower than you think it should be, check the composition of your contraceptive pill and ask your doctor to change it if it contains too much progesterone.

There are two possible downsides to taking male hormones. Too much can give you facial hair and other unwanted male sexual characteristics. However, this does not usually happen with the correct dose. The second potential complication is not dose-related: The added testosterone may raise the cholesterol level, decrease the good fraction (HDL), and increase the harmful kind (LDL). So if you have severe risk factors for heart disease such as a bad family history, high cholesterol, elevated blood pressure, or diabetes, monitor your blood fats while taking testosterone supplements.

High blood pressure, whether treated or not, can interfere with a woman's libido. Among some 200 women with untreated hypertension, a significant number reported diminished and delayed orgasm, vaginal dryness, and painful intercourse. Many commonly used drugs to lower pressure can also impair libido. You may have to experiment with several such agents before you find one that can normalize your high pressure yet leave you feeling sexy.

It's commonly believed that in men of a "certain" age, a lack of testosterone is the cause of a decline in their sex drive. That's why so many of them take testosterone supplements in the form of pills, patches, injections, and creams (lathered on a flaccid penis), all in search of their lost libido. These maneuvers are usually in vain because testosterone levels do not fall as dramatically in aging men as estrogen does in menopausal women, and a lack of testosterone is not usually why male libido declines with age. In fact, only 20 to 25 percent of cases of diminished libido are due to hormonal factors.

Extra testosterone when you've got enough of your own is no more effective than a placebo, but, unlike a placebo, such supplements can hurt you. Testosterone is made by the testes under the supervision and control of the pituitary and hypothalamus glands in the brain. When these glands sense that there's enough testosterone circulating in the bloodstream, they signal the testes to stop their production—until the testosterone level falls again. When you take supplemental testosterone by whatever route, it gets into the bloodstream, fools the brain into thinking that you've got plenty of your own, and so the testes are directed to cut back their production. If they remain inactive for long enough, they begin to shrink, atrophy, and lose their ability to make testosterone. In that case, you may end up with nice large breasts, the envy of every woman on your block. This is only one of the risks of extra testosterone when your natural supply is adequate. There are others: Testosterone supplements can damage your liver, raise your cholesterol level, and, according to many specialists, promote cancer of the prostate by activating dormant malignant cells lying deep inside the prostate.

The best way to determine whether you're testosterone deficient is to measure its level in the blood. That's a routine test available in most laboratories. If you are truly low in testosterone (normal range is from 300 to 1,200 nanograms per deciliter of blood), there are several ways to increase it: by injection, orally, or topically. The easiest, most effective, and safest way is the skin patch (marketed as Testoderm and Androderm), which releases testosterone more evenly and gradually than do the oral or injection routes. The older preparations of these patches had to be applied to the scrotum; those currently available can be placed anywhere—on the back, abdomen, thigh, or upper arm.

How to Cope with a Failing Libido

Men and women with a waning sex drive should first identify and correct any hormonal deficiencies. But keep in mind that there are many physical reasons for a lack of interest in sex. For example.

• **Review with your doctor each and every medicine or herb you're taking.** Antidepressants, especially the selective serotonin uptake inhibitors such as Prozac, can reduce sexual desire. So can many blood pressure–lowering drugs, especially the beta-blockers—propranolol (Inderal), atenolol (Tenormin), metoprolol

(Lopressor), and others. If they are compromising your sex drive, you may have to reduce their dosage or switch to some other agent.

• **Which comes first, the chicken or the egg?** Are you depressed because you've lost your sex drive or is your libido low because you're depressed? In my opinion, depression is more often responsible for a waning sex life than all other causes combined. You owe it to yourself and your partner to check it out. Treating depression is the best way to restore libido in such cases.

• **If you have zero libido and are taking "recreational" drugs,** or even suspect you have a drinking problem, don't expect hormones to fix matters until you go on the wagon.

• **If you've had a heart attack** and are afraid that the stress of sex will endanger your health, discuss your anxiety with your doctor. (This also applies to wives, whose own libido may be suppressed because they're afraid that sex will hurt their husbands.) Generally speaking, if you can walk up two flights of stairs comfortably (elevators don't count), lovemaking won't harm you. Your physical ability to have sex can be easily determined by having one of several kinds of stress tests available in most doctors' offices and hospitals.

• **If you've been avoiding sex because you're tired** and just don't feel up to it, get a thorough physical exam. Correcting anemia or eradicating a low-grade infection is much more likely to restore your libido than is taking any hormone supplement arbitrarily.

• **If you're a woman, don't accept your partner's**

impotence as inevitable, and then rationalize your own passivity to it by concluding that you're "too old" for it anyway. There are many ways to treat male impotence these days. (See Chapter 7.)

• **If you've lost your spouse,** keep alive the memories of the wonderful times you had together but don't dwell on them. There's nothing worse than loneliness, and no number of children or other family members will cure it. Keep an open mind on making new friendships, particularly with the opposite sex. Remember that people who were once happily married are the most likely to remarry or form new "friendships" after their spouses have passed on. And you're never too old to do so.

• **"Use it or lose it":** I can't think of a single area in medicine where this adage is more appropriate than in the matter of sex and libido. Regular sex, whether alone or in concert, helps your sex organs continue to function normally. This is especially true in women. The more sexually active you are, the more flexible, elastic, and moist your vagina will be. Abstinence, enforced or by preference, causes the vaginal tissues to atrophy or shrink. This can render sex unpleasant and painful.

• **If estrogen replacement therapy,** and especially vaginal estrogen creams, don't provide sufficient lubrication, there are several jellies you can use. My patients prefer K-Y Jelly, Astroglide, Replens, and, when itching is a problem, vitamin E cream. Ask your gynecologist for other suggestions. Avoid products that provoke an allergic reaction, and keep away from deodorant soaps and various hygiene sprays that dry your tissues and irritate them. When the vagina loses its natural acidity as you grow older, yeast and other infections can develop more easily. Dry yourself thoroughly after a shower or bath, because bacteria and fungi thrive on damp skin. Cotton underwear breathes better and is less likely to retain moisture than nylon or silk. Also, empty your bladder immediately after sex to reduce the chances of infection.

• **Men and women who exercise regularly usually have the best and most active sex lives.** In addition to helping you feel better, exercise results in increased blood flow to the pelvic area where, as you probably know, the key sex organs are located.

• **Age sometimes causes the muscles that support the vagina, uterus, and bladder to relax.** The cervix may then slip into the vagina, making intercourse painful. Such prolapse can often be corrected surgically, or treated with various support devices. If you develop incontinence, especially when you strain, cough, or sneeze, ask your gynecologist to teach you how to do the Kegel exercises. They not only improve incontinence, they help the vagina contract, and provide greater pleasure to you and your partner during sex.

• **Women cannot prevent menopause** or raise their estrogen level without taking replacement therapy, but men can increase their testosterone level by weight lifting. However, too much exercise and not enough rest will drop the testosterone level—as well as the libido. If your testosterone concentration is low and you're a vegetarian, have a steak now and then. Meat eaters generally have more circulating testosterone than do vegetarians.

- **There are several methods, and more are on the way, to help impotent men whose libido is still pretty good** (see Chapter 7). But if your libido is wanting, ask your doctor about an aphrodisiac from Sweden that's currently being tested in this country. It's called, appropriately enough, Libido, and is made from the components of fertilized, partly incubated chicken eggs. Double-blind crossover studies have shown it to improve sexual desire within two weeks in 58 percent of men. In other reports, the response rate was as high as 80 percent. The dosage is 3 grams taken twice a day. It's been found to be most effective when the drop in libido is due to such antidepressants as Prozac. No important side effects have been reported.

What to Remember about Lack of Libido

1. Aging doesn't necessarily mean the end of your sex life. If your libido has lessened, discuss the problem with your doctor and make sure that no other underlying medical condition is causing it. Try to identify other reasons, such as some treatable disease, medication, depression, or alcohol and substance abuse.
2. Hormone deficiency in both sexes, as we get older, does play a part in libido reduction, but it's not the whole story. However, estrogen replacement usually helps, mostly by acting on female sex organs so that intercourse is pleasurable, not painful. In some

cases, however, estrogens are not enough, and menopausal women may require male-hormone (testosterone) supplements to restore a flagging sex drive.

3. Lack of testosterone in men as a cause of their diminished libido is greatly exaggerated. Too many take supplements unnecessarily and without benefit. Testosterone can result in several side effects, including prostate cancer and ultimately, believe it or not, in feminization.

4. Exercise and a healthy lifestyle enhance well-being and improve one's sex drive.

10

MENOPAUSE

His and Hers

When I was ten or eleven years old, I became aware of a change in my mother's behavior. One didn't have to be a doctor, a medical student, or even an adult to know that she wasn't her usual happy self. Always outgoing and warm, she now seemed nervous, uptight, and impatient with my father and me. There were times when she didn't say a word at dinner, and she often cried for no apparent reason. From time to time, even in the middle of winter, she'd perspire profusely and throw open a window—this in frigid Montreal! I also noticed that her face would suddenly become red and flushed, even when she wasn't angry or embarrassed.

One day, as our family doctor was leaving after making a house call (Mother had asked him to come because she wasn't feeling well), I overheard him telling my father that she was having trouble with her "changes." I loved my mother and was very worried about her. I wanted to know what these "changes" were; I needed to be reassured that she was okay. So I asked my father what it was all about. He said he really couldn't explain it, but implied that her "changes" were beyond her control and that there was nothing anyone could do about them.

She continued acting this way for about two years. Then, shortly after my bar mitzvah celebration, Mom was suddenly her old self again—no more crying, no more flushing, no more sweating—happy as a lark. I couldn't understand why her "changes" had changed.

It wasn't until I took a high-school course in biology that I learned about menopause, that it was synonymous with "changes," and that "changes" was short for "change of life"—when a woman's periods end. The word *menopause* comes from "pause in the menses," but why "change of life"?

To this day, I haven't gotten a satisfactory answer to that question. The most common explanation is that life changes when the ovaries slow down their production of estrogen and progesterone, when they no longer send eggs down the fallopian tubes to unite with sperm, when the periods end, when a woman can no longer have babies and doesn't need prophylactic contraceptives anymore. If that's the case, why isn't it called change of life or menopause in a woman who's had her uterus removed but whose ovaries are intact? Her periods have ended too, she also can't have children, and no longer needs contraceptives.

The answer, of course, is that the central feature of menopause is the altered hormonal status. That's what changes so many aspects of life. Symptoms vary from woman to woman, as does vulnerability to a host of biological changes and medical disorders. But all menopausal females have in common a marked decline in the production and availability of the hormones that affected every one of their body organs and functions since puberty: the reproductive and urinary tracts, the heart and blood vessels, bones, breasts, skin, hair, pelvic muscles, and brain.

Menopause Defined

By definition, menopause is a natural process that causes symptoms starting around age forty-five and increasing in intensity for months or years until the periods end, usually by age fifty-one. They may, however, continue until age fifty-five. (I have seen thirty-five-year-old women who were menopausal, and some who continued to menstruate well into their fifties. Menopause is considered to be "premature" when it occurs naturally before age forty-five.) The interval between the earliest onset of the symptoms and the time the menses (periods) finally end is called *perimenopause*. It is characterized by a progressive increase in severity of the symptoms described below.

Menopause is not something of which a woman suddenly becomes aware when she wakes up one morning. It evolves gradually as ovarian secretion of hormones declines. Bleeding becomes irregular and the periods shorter, until they eventually end. (Caution: Let your doctor know about any change in your menstrual pattern. Bleeding between periods or a heavier flow at any age should be considered abnormal until proven otherwise. Don't assume that these symptoms are due to menopause simply because you're in your late forties. There are many other possible and unrelated causes.)

Menopause has officially arrived when, for no other reason, you haven't had a period for twelve consecutive months. (Don't confuse natural menopause with one that's induced by removal of the ovaries. Here, symptoms set in more abruptly and they are usually more severe. Drugs and radiation therapy can also damage the ovaries and cause premature menopause. Whatever the mechanism, the end result is the same: no hormones.)

Remember that you may still be fertile during the first year after your periods have ended, so continue to use contraceptives. The world is full of surprised, not-so-young mothers in their late forties who abandoned birth-control measures because they were sure their childbearing days were over. Taking a contraceptive pill in this twilight zone of fertility will usually alleviate some of your menopausal symptoms since it contains an even higher biological equivalent of estrogen than the usual hormone replacement therapy. But the pill is not for you if you smoke, currently have breast cancer, or are at special risk for heart disease because of high blood pressure, too much cholesterol, diabetes, or the other factors discussed in Chapter 6, "Heart Attack."

Menopause Myths

I learned a lot more about menopause in medical school than I did in my first biology class, but not all of what I learned was accurate. The subject is still shrouded in folklore even in the hallowed halls of medical learning. For example, I'll bet you think that the younger you were when your periods started, the later your menopause; that if you are underweight, you will have an earlier menopause; that how old you are when your periods stop in some way depends on the number of children you've had and whether or not you took oral contraceptives. I don't believe any of these associations. But here are some valid ones: If you're a smoker, or even a former one, your menopause will start earlier than if you'd never smoked. Periods end about three years earlier in women smokers. There is also a genetic component: You're likely to go through menopause at about the same age as your mother and grandmother. Also, if you've had a hysterectomy but your ovaries were spared, menopause is apt to set in earlier.

Symptoms of Menopause

• **Hot flashes:** The hot flush or flash is the hallmark symptom of menopause. It occurs in 50 to 75 percent of women. In the typical attack, the skin turns pink, sweat breaks out on your face, your back, or the front of your chest; you feel warm and your heart pounds. These symptoms usually last one to three minutes and are frequently followed by a chill; they may occur several times a day or only occasionally; they can be spontaneous or, more likely, happen when you're overheated, drinking alcohol, caffeine, hot liquids, eating spicy foods, or in the midst of a stressful situation. What precipitates a hot flash, as well as its severity and duration, varies from woman to woman, but every female's pattern is consistent and predictable.

Drenching perspiration, another characteristic symptom of menopausal women, interrupts their normal sleep pattern, leaving them tired and irritable the next day (much as does sleep apnea).

Hot flashes may come and go for just a few months, or continue for as long as five years or more. Although they are not a threat to life, they are uncomfortable and inconvenient. It didn't make much difference to my mother when she flushed, flashed, and perspired in my presence, but women in senior positions in government, industry, and other professions can find such attacks embarrassing. Imagine suddenly flushing and perspiring while performing delicate surgery, or conducting a press briefing as attorney general, or being secretary of state and negotiating with a head of state, or as a CEO laying down the law at an important meeting (attended by men!).

Hot flashes are the result of estrogen deficiency. The body normally stabilizes its temperature very efficiently. This regulating system is controlled by the hypothalamus in the brain, whose function is affected by estrogen. When the estrogen supply drops, the hypothalamus responds by releasing certain hormones that quickly raise body temperature and cause a hot flash. These symptoms are said to reflect vasomotor instability, dilatation, and constriction of blood vessels.

Estrogen supplements prevent hot flashes or make them much less severe. But if you choose not to take them, you should wear light, layered, cotton clothing, especially in the summer, and drink some ice water at the very onset of the attack. Some women feel better when they avoid chocolate, alcohol, and caffeine. Catapres (clonidine), a blood pressure–lowering pill, often helps prevent these attacks, but I don't usually prescribe it because it can be associated with too many side effects, especially dizziness and fatigue. It may also cause withdrawal symptoms when discontinued abruptly.

• **Vaginal dryness:** When deprived of estrogen, the vagina becomes dry, shorter, narrower, and its lining thins and is prone to infection, irritation, and urinary incontinence. Under these circumstances, intercourse causes more pain than pleasure. But don't let that deter you, because maintaining a high level of sexual activity, even under these adverse conditions, minimizes the long-term wasting (atrophy) of the vaginal walls. Here are some palliative measures to improve matters: Use a water-based lubricant such as K-Y Jelly or vaginal moisturizing creams such as Replens (available without a prescription); engage in foreplay a little longer so as to increase vaginal moisture; learn how to strengthen the tone of your fragile vaginal muscles to enhance your sexual pleasure and to prevent urinary incontinence.

These voluntary contractions of the pelvic and the uro-genital muscles are called Kegel exercises. Your gyne-cologist or a good physiotherapist can teach you how to do them. All these steps help, but they are not nearly as effective as hormonal supplements that you can take by mouth, in a skin patch, or as a vaginal cream. The latter therapy works quickly, in a matter of weeks; the pill and patch take several months to restore normal vaginal moisture.

• **Urinary incontinence:** Urinary incontinence is a common and embarrassing symptom that affects 25 to 50 percent of all menopausal women. As is the case in the vagina, when there is less estrogen available, the lining of the urinary tract also becomes thin. The pelvic muscles that control bladder function are weakened too. The ure-thra (the tube that carries urine from the bladder) loses the pressure necessary to prevent your urine from leaking out of the body. So when you sneeze, cough, laugh, or ex-ercise, you wet yourself.

Although urinary incontinence can be improved by strengthening the pelvic muscles with the Kegel or simi-lar exercises, hormone replacement is more effective. Es-trogen increases muscle strength and tone by improving the circulation to the organs in the pelvic area. If that doesn't help, and the exercises don't work, and you find yourself living with a diaper or a pad, ask your doctor about correcting the problem surgically.

• **Sagging breasts:** Sagging breasts are the plague of many menopausal women. Breasts sag because their glandular tissue is replaced by fat; the bigger the breasts, the greater the sag. The only thing you can do to minimize sagging is hormone therapy, which slows down the replacement of supportive glandular tissue by fat. (However, estrogen also causes a proliferation of the duct system in the breasts and is probably the reason for the sensation of fullness that some women feel on this therapy.) Exercises don't help because there are no muscles to firm up in the breast. If hormone replacements don't stop the process and you're unhappy about your appearance, you can have cosmetic surgery.

• **Hair changes:** In some women, the decreased estrogen of menopause results in a relative increase of testosterone, the male hormone. This darkens and thickens body and facial hair, and thins your scalp and pubic hair. You can deal with these changes in several ways, the most effective being hormone replacement. However, you can also have electrolysis, pluck the hair out yourself, or use a hair-removal cream.

• **Aging skin:** If you've been a sun worshiper for any length of time, your skin is apt to sag and wrinkle. Cigarette smoking makes matters worse. Lack of estrogen is the final coup de grâce. At menopause, your skin becomes thinner and less elastic since the body produces less collagen, the stuff that supports the skin. I've discussed how best to manage these changes in Chapter 14, "Aging Skin." Suffice it to say that hormone replacement tends to maintain normal skin thickness and enhance the body's production of collagen.

• **Mood changes:** Have you noticed that your moods have changed along with your periods? Are you depressed and irritable? Do you have trouble concentrating? Is a good night's sleep only a memory? Don't rush to blame all this on your hormones. Some of life's other difficulties may be making you feel this way. If hormone replacement doesn't solve the problem, think about getting some counseling or psychological support.

• **Lack of libido:** Waning hormone production can affect your sex drive. If estrogen replacement therapy does not restore your passion, ask your doctor for a small amount of male hormone (but not enough to grow a beard).

• **Osteoporosis:** Osteoporosis, the disorder in which the bones lose calcium, become thin, and break easily, is the cause of many deaths and much disability among postmenopausal women. Earlier in life, the calcium we eat is stored in the bones and kept there by estrogen. When the ovaries decrease their estrogen production, calcium is no longer deposited in bone, and what's already there begins to seep out. (This is more fully discussed in Chapter 12, "Osteoporosis.") The strategy for preventing osteoporosis consists of reversing all these mechanisms. Ideally, then, a menopausal woman should take estrogen, continue to consume enough calcium (either in her diet or from supplements), have enough exposure to sunlight for her skin to make the vitamin D that bones require, and engage in ongoing exercise. Being underweight, smoking, or drinking more than modest amounts of alcohol all aggravate osteoporosis.

Instead of estrogen, there are now several other effective agents to retard osteoporosis. These include Fosamax, calcitonin, long-acting sodium fluoride, and raloxifene (Evista).

• **Heart disease:** Before menopause, women are protected from heart attacks by their female hormones. When estrogen levels drop, cholesterol increases, and there is less of the good HDL and more of the undesirable LDL. These changes promote plaque formation and ultimate closure of the coronary arteries. Estrogen supplements delay this process by lowering cholesterol, raising the HDL, and reducing the LDL. However, it appears that starting estrogen replacement *after* a woman has developed heart disease may be dangerous. In my own practice, I do not usually prescribe hormone replacement therapy to menopausal women with heart disease. However, if you've been taking estrogen all along and are found to have heart disease, don't stop the hormones abruptly. Discuss with your doctor the pros and cons of continuing it.

Taking estrogen is not a license for abandoning common sense. Blood fats are only one risk factor for heart disease, although an important one. To protect yourself, you must also do something about elevated blood pressure, high sugar levels if you're diabetic, overweight, physical inactivity, cigarette smoking, and stress.

One of the main reasons so many women won't take estrogen is the fear that it promotes cancer, notably of the breast and uterus. That fear is justified to some extent, but supplemental estrogen also reduces the risk of heart disease, a much bigger killer than any cancer. The bottom line is that women who take estrogen live longer and better. (See Chapter 2, "Cancer," and Chapter 6, "Heart Attacks.")

• **Diabetes:** Diabetes is the latest addition to the roster of disorders that are either prevented or improved by estrogen supplements. In a recent large study of more than 14,000 menopausal women with the adult-onset form of the disease, those who took estrogen had lower blood sugars than those who didn't. And five times as many women who did not take estrogen developed diabetes than those who did.

It's not clear why estrogen has such a favorable effect on blood sugar. Most researchers think that it probably reduces the body's insulin resistance, and so improves the way it handles sugar.

On the basis of these data, it's reasonable for any menopausal woman with a family history of diabetes to consider hormone supplements. Also, since African Americans and Hispanics are at greater statistical risk for diabetes, they too should give serious thought to all the advantages of taking estrogen after menopause.

Easing the Symptoms of Menopause

There are three sex hormones whose production drops dramatically with menopause: estrogen, progesterone, and testosterone. A drop in the concentration of any of them may produce symptoms. Overall, however, the main hormonal player in the menopause game is estrogen. If you still have your uterus, you must take some progesterone along with estrogen because the latter alone (or, as doctors refer to it, "unopposed") leaves you significantly more prone to uterine cancer. Progesterone reduces that risk. However, if you've had a hysterectomy, do not take the additional progesterone. (Estrogen replacement alone is referred to as ERT; when any other hormone is added to the regimen, it's called hormone replacement therapy, or HRT.) For convenience' sake, I will use the term HRT whenever referring to menopausal hormonal replacement therapy.

HRT—THE PROS AND CONS

Replacing the missing hormones not only eases or eradicates the troublesome symptoms of menopause but, more important, it also reduces the risk of osteoporosis, stroke, heart attack, Alzheimer's, and other manifestations of aging. However, only a fraction of women take them because most menopausal symptoms become less severe with time and eventually disappear. Many women prefer to wait them out rather than take hormones that have side effects and can cause cancer of the uterus and probably of the breast, too. But remember that even though the symptoms clear up, the increased risk of several serious diseases due to lack of estrogen does not.

Every woman must decide for herself whether or not to take HRT based on her own health profile. For example, if you have a strong family history of breast cancer, you may prefer not to take something that can increase your already substantial risk for developing it yourself. On the other hand, if you have several documented risk factors for heart attack you may be willing to take your chances with cancer or put up with the troublesome side effects of HRT described below. By the same token, if you've already had one bone fracture and densitometry reveals that you are a candidate for another, you may prefer to cope with the adverse effects of HRT in order to reap its benefits.

Despite all the advantages of HRT, it's not a free ride. Here are some of the more important risks and side effects:

- Endometrial (uterine) cancer. If you still have your uterus, always take additional progesterone along with the estrogen to reduce this possibility.
- Gallbladder disease requiring surgery is more common in menopausal women who take estrogen.
- Estrogen and progesterone can result in a host of symptomatic side effects that include nausea and vomiting, painful enlargement of the breasts, and fluid retention, all of which can in turn aggravate other existing conditions, such as asthma, epilepsy, migraine, and kidney or heart disease.
- Progesterone often results in the return of the "periods," and even PMS, from which you thought you were finally emancipated.
- The possibility of hormone-induced breast cancer, though not proven to everyone's satisfaction, remains

a real threat of which you should be aware, especially if there is a strong family history for it.

- Unopposed estrogen—that is, without added progesterone—may also lead to spasm of the arteries. This shows up as the Raynaud phenomenon, in which the tips of the fingers, nose, and even the earlobes become blue and painful when exposed to cold. This is because the little arteries that supply them become constricted. Such spasm may also account for other vascular disorders from which menopausal women suffer: migraine headaches, angina due to the temporary contraction of the coronary arteries (Prinzmetal's angina), and even an elevated pressure in the lungs (pulmonary hypertension). None of these abnormalities occur when progesterone is added to estrogen. If you have Raynaud's, migraines, or some unexplained lung disorder and are taking estrogen alone because your uterus was removed, discuss the matter with your doctor. It may be wise to add progesterone to prevent the spasm disorder.

All of the above notwithstanding, I am keen on HRT because its benefits outweigh its risks and side effects. And by the way, once started, I am of the opinion that it should be continued indefinitely. Its advantages extend into the advanced years. Doctors like me who push for it, especially if they're male, are sometimes accused of viewing menopause as if it were a disease rather than a natural female biological event. Those opposed to HRT ask why we should burden essentially healthy women with the cost, inconvenience, and side effects of a med-

ication for the rest of their lives. Although they concede
that estrogen does protect against heart disease and that
those who take it do live longer and better, they point out,
quite correctly, that adding progesterone to the replacement regimen reduces these protective cardiac effects (it
may reduce them, but does not nullify them).

Those who are opposed to the use of estrogen emphasize the risk that estrogen poses for cancer of the breast.
That risk probably does exist, although some doctors remain unconvinced. However, death and disability from
heart disease, broken hips, and other bone fractures far
outweigh the morbidity and mortality of breast cancer. If
you're taking estrogen and are worried about breast cancer, have yourself examined twice a year and be sure to
take an annual mammogram. However, if you have a
strong genetic risk, or if you have the BrCa1 or BrCa2
genes, you should not be on HRT. These genes reflect an
increased vulnerability to breast cancer, and women with
a strong family history for this malignancy are often en-
couraged to be tested for their presence.

Estrogen Preparations

Walk into any drugstore and you'll be surprised by how
many brands of estrogen there are, and the number of
ways you can take them: tablets, injectables, creams,
patches, pellets, and vaginal inserts. Which one to use,
and in what dosage, depends on your specific needs and
preferences. Competition among pharmaceutical houses

being what it is and given the fact that patents on every drug do run out, there are always some "me too" products of every medication. However, the variety of these estrogen preparations may reflect the fact that women are constantly looking for more acceptable ones. So find the product that best suits you.

The most widely used tablets include:

Conjugated estrogens (Premarin), available in four different dosages, ranging from 0.3 to 1.25 milligrams. This product is probably the best known and most widely used form of estrogen replacement, the "gold standard" for many women and doctors. Start with the lowest dose and increase it gradually over a period of weeks or months, depending on your response. The most usual maintenance dose is 0.625 milligrams, but you may need more if your ovaries were surgically removed. Premarin is made from *pre*gnant *mar*es' ur*ine*.

Estradiol (Estrace) is an estrogen that's favored by many gynecologists and their patients because it is micronized and thus well absorbed from the intestinal tract. It comes in three strengths: 0.58, 1.0, and 2.0 milligrams.

Other brand names, among which there appears to be little difference, are Ogen, Estratab, and Estinyl. The latter is used more for oral contraception than for simple estrogen replacement.

Topical estrogen is becoming increasingly more popular. It's absorbed from the skin and goes directly into the bloodstream, bypassing the liver. These patches are especially useful if you cannot tolerate oral estrogen or don't absorb it well, or if you have liver disease. The earlier preparations often irritated the skin, especially in hot weather, but the newer ones are much improved. You can either get the one-a-week strength or the two-a-week strength. Although changing the patch once a week is more convenient, it does become soiled, and many women prefer to replace it twice weekly. A 0.05-milligram patch is biologically equivalent to 0.625 milligrams of Premarin.

There are several different brands of patches, the most popular of which are estradiol marketed as Vivelle and Climara. However, there is another estradiol preparation called Estradose made in France and available in this country. I learned about it from several patients, and have been recommending it to others. It's a transdermal gel that has the advantage of being absorbed almost immediately after it's applied. This eliminates an unsightly patch that becomes soiled and causes skin irritation.

Estrogen can also be administered by injection at intervals of about three weeks. This is an alternative for women who prefer not to take the daily tablets or wear the patches. The problem with injections is that the estrogen level is initially very high, but then drops. Thus, you may begin to develop symptoms several days before the next injection is due.

If you're having urinary problems or vaginal dryness, Premarin and Estrace are available as vaginal creams that act locally and more quickly than the oral preparations. Estring is a newer way to deliver estrogen vaginally. It's a Silastic ring the size of a diaphragm that contains estrogen and can be left in place for as long as three months.

Vaginal preparations help local symptoms, but because their absorption is unpredictable, they do not have the same impact as oral estrogen on the prevention of the more serious consequences of estrogen deficiency.

Your doctor can place estrogen pellets under the skin with a needle every three or four months. Though used in Europe, the FDA has not approved them at the time of writing. Their major drawback is the fact that they cannot be removed once they've been inserted.

How can you tell whether your estrogen supplement is working? Mainly by the way you feel. However, your doctor can determine its effect by examining samples of your vaginal tissue under a microscope to see if the cells are estrogen-deprived, or by measuring hormone levels in the blood.

Progesterone Preparations

The ovaries make progesterone in the last half of the menstrual cycle. Estrogen replacement without progesterone increases the risk of cancer of the lining of the uterus. If you are menopausal and still have your uterus and are taking HRT, you must add progesterone.

There are two forms of this hormone available in the United States: progesterone and progestin. The best known brands of progesterone, Provera and Amen, come in 2.5-, 5.0-, and 10-milligram tablets. Some doctors prefer progestin because they believe it is more predictably absorbed. Progesterone supplements are either taken daily in small doses along with the estrogen, or in higher doses for the last ten days of the month.

Testosterone Preparations

Remember that the ovaries make small amounts of testosterone along with the normal complement of estrogen and progesterone. The ovaries and the adrenal glands (sitting atop the kidneys, where they also produce adrenaline and the cortisone-type hormones) make other male hormones (androgens) in women.

The relatively small amount of testosterone produced in the ovary has specific effects in women: It gives them energy, stimulates their libido, enlarges the clitoris, increases muscle mass, and enhances appetite. After menopause, the ovaries cut down their production of all three hormones—estrogen, progesterone, and testosterone. The resulting diminished sex drive and lack of energy can often be corrected by adding testosterone supplements to the usual HRT. However, be careful not to take too much. There's rarely a reason for dosages higher than 2.5 milligrams of methyltestosterone a day. If you take more than that, you're likely to develop such masculinizing side effects as too much hair in the wrong places; weight gain; coarse, oily skin with acne; a bigger clitoris than you want; and a lower pitch to your voice. Be especially careful with these male supplements if you already have high cholesterol or a high-risk profile for heart disease, because testosterone raises cholesterol and acts adversely on its HDL and LDL fractions.

Testosterone comes in tablets (often combined with Premarin or some other estrogen), by injection (either alone or in combination with female hormones), or as a cream. Patches are widely used by men but should not be taken by women because their dosage is too high. Pellets in a 75-milligram strength are approved by the FDA, and can be implanted every three or four months. They are taken in addition to HRT. The advantage of testosterone by this route is that it doesn't go through the liver, and so has less of a harmful HDL-lowering effect.

Phytoestrogens

There has been an explosion of interest in "natural" substitutes and nutrients to replace synthetic drugs and hormones for the prevention and treatment of disease. Some of these substances, called phytoestrogens, are very popular substitutes for estrogen in the management of menopausal symptoms. Phytoestrogens in the diet come mainly from fruits, vegetables, and meat. The two that have been most intensively studied in humans are lignans (from the breakdown by intestinal bacteria of grains, fibers, flaxseed, fruits, and vegetables) and isoflavones, which are present in soybeans and other legumes.

When estrogen acts on an organ anywhere in the body, it does so by attaching itself to that organ at a specific site where "receptor" cells make the actual binding possible.

Phytoestrogens are compounds produced by many plants. They are unique in that they compete with estrogen at these receptor sites. When an estrogen molecule comes along and wants to sit down on a receptor, it finds that its "natural" cousin, the phytoestrogen, is already there. The weaker phytoestrogen takes over the job of providing the hormonelike actions.

One of the arguments in favor of using phytoestrogens for menopausal women is the observation that Asian women who eat lots of soy foods rich in phytoestrogens have fewer menopausal symptoms (although they have a higher incidence of osteoporosis). They also have less breast cancer and heart disease, a very compelling epidemiological statistic. When these women migrate to the West, those who adopt our diet and abandon the Asian diet apparently lose these benefits.

Phytoestrogens are big business in this country. The most popular products are dong quai (*Angelica sinensis*), black cohosh, soy in various forms, and flaxseed. Dong quai has powerful pharmacological properties and estrogenlike effects and has been used for centuries in oriental medicine. Some Western pharmacologists, however, caution against its use. They worry about the potential toxicity of several of its active ingredients, such as coumarins and safrole, the latter being a component of dong quai's essential oils.

Black cohosh, on the other hand, appears to be effective and safe. The complementary medical literature contains many references to its usefulness in controlling hot flashes, and it may even possess inhibitory effects on estrogen-dependent cancers (of the breast, ovaries, and uterus). Unlike progesterone, it appears to have a beneficial effect on cholesterol levels. It's sold in health-food stores as Remifemin. If you're going to try any of these phytoestrogens, this one is probably your best bet, along with soy and flaxseed products.

Male Menopause

Of course it's possible! Why else would the first three letters of menopause spell "men"?

Doctors who believe that there is such a thing as male menopause (admittedly a minority) say that it occurs in about 40 percent of men between the ages of forty-five and sixty. Its main symptoms are:

- Depression
- Feelings of inadequacy and hopelessness
- Irritability
- Lethargy
- Mood swings
- Insomnia
- Headaches
- Loss of concentration
- Weight gain (a paunch) and simultaneous loss of muscle
- Impaired memory
- Decreased libido and impaired sexual performance
- Diminished stamina
- Difficulty making decisions

This constellation of symptoms is said to explain the seven-year itch—why some men abandon their wives and run off with younger women, spend a fortune on snazzy sports cars, and have other manifestations of the "midlife crisis."

If there is a male menopause, is it due to lack of testosterone? Should that hormone be measured in all middle-aged men and then replaced if necessary? Most doctors don't think so. They believe that this stereotypical midlife crisis is more likely due to psychological causes: the fear of aging and mortality as men see parents and friends die, marital problems, the realization that many of their ambitions will never be fulfilled, and depression as their kids leave home. There are also physical reasons that have nothing to do with hormones: an alcohol habit that's finally caught up with them, untreated high blood pressure, cigarette smoking, self-medication with who-knows-what drugs for who-knows-what symptoms, lack of exercise, or circulatory problems.

Everyone agrees that at this time in their lives, men should review their overall lifestyle and make the appropriate changes, such as trying to reduce chronic stress; quitting smoking; watching their diet with particular reference to cholesterol, fat, and salt; exercising regularly; and having an annual checkup.

If you're developing the symptoms listed above, ask your doctor for a testosterone blood analysis. A waning testosterone supply can have debilitating effects. However, although levels do drop after age forty-five, the significance and impact of this fall are not clear, since many men with reduced levels are perfectly well.

One explanation for the variation in behavior observed with different levels of testosterone may be the form in which that hormone is present. Testosterone can either be free or attached to protein. The bound testosterone is neutralized; free testosterone, on the other hand, is the active form responsible for masculinity, energy, libido, the handsome beard, and all the other characteristics of which men are so proud. A routine testosterone analysis does not distinguish between these two forms of the hormone.

If you're not feeling right and your free testosterone level is borderline or lower, try supplements. There are studies documenting improvement not only in sexual function, but also in muscle strength and general well-being in men whose low testosterone hormone levels have been restored to a normal-to-high range.

As is the case with female hormones, you can take the missing testosterone in several ways: orally, by shots, patches, or pellets. The oral form can hurt the liver. If you choose injections, you'll need them every two weeks to maintain an optimal hormonal level; implants are placed surgically in your gluteus muscle (what you sit on) and you'll need a new pellet every three or four months. Most men prefer the transdermal patch, which is changed daily.

Like estrogen, testosterone replacement has its downside. So think twice about these supplements even if you appear to need them. The most common side effect is weight gain, but there are other, more worrisome consequences. High doses have been reported to cause heart attacks and strokes, especially in younger men. The complication that concerns me most is the possibility that extra testosterone may activate dormant cancer cells in the prostate gland and cause them to multiply and spread. So stay away from these supplements if you have prostate cancer. Remember that the basic therapy for this malignancy is to neutralize whatever testosterone is present. You're also better off avoiding these supplements even if your prostate is benignly enlarged, if you have sleep apnea, or if your blood is "thick."

What to Remember about Menopause

1. Menopause in women refers to the decrease in the amount of hormones produced by the ovaries.
2. The ovaries make three hormones—estrogen, progesterone, and testosterone—all of which contribute to the symptoms of consequences of menopause.
3. Menopause is a gradual process that continues for a period of months or years before the periods stop. This interval is known as perimenopause. Menopause has arrived when you've had no periods for twelve months.
4. Some women remain fertile during perimenopause, so this is no time to stop taking contraceptives.
5. Symptoms of menopause vary in nature and severity from woman to woman, but they are consistent in each individual.

6. Although most menopausal symptoms, such as hot flashes, gradually become less severe and clear up in two years or less, they may persist much longer.

7. The major consequences of menopause are increased vulnerability to heart disease, osteoporosis, and stroke.

8. Estrogen replacement effectively controls symptoms of menopause but, more important, it reduces the risk of the serious complications of lack of estrogen.

9. Estrogen increases the risk of uterine cancer. Women who have not had a hysterectomy must take progesterone along with estrogen to prevent that complication.

10. Progesterone may compromise some of the beneficial effects of estrogen, especially vis-à-vis heart disease, and cause the return of "periods."

11. Lack of libido in menopausal women is more likely due to a decrease in the testosterone levels than to lack of estrogen, the replacement of which may not solve the problem.

12. Estrogen has been implicated as a cause of breast cancer, although there's no definite proof as yet. Women who are vulnerable to breast cancer should consult their doctors before starting hormonal supplements.

13. All women on hormonal supplements should have annual mammograms and semiannual breast examinations.

14. Estrogen can be taken by mouth, by injection, in the vagina as a cream, or topically in a patch.

15. The concept of a male menopause is not universally accepted.

16. The symptoms of midlife crisis experienced by some 40 percent of men between the ages of forty-five and sixty may be due to nonhormonal problems, to a decrease in testosterone production by the testes, or to a combination of both.

17. If lack of testosterone is suspected, its levels can be measured in the blood.

18. Testosterone supplements can be taken orally, by injection, by pellet implant, or transdermally. The latter is currently the most popular method of administration.

19. Testosterone may precipitate vascular problems in younger men, and should never be taken by anyone with cancer or enlargement of the prostate gland.

11

OSTEOARTHRITIS

A Joint Declaration

Some 40 million Americans have arthritis—that's one in every six. It's the most prevalent chronic health problem and the number-one cause of pain and limitation of movement in this country. If you were to accost at random twelve people over the age of fifty anywhere in America and ask them if they have "arthritis," some would tell you it's none of your business and a few would report you to a cop for harassing them, but at least two would say yes. If any of them happened to be a rheumatologist, he or she would probably ask you what kind of arthritis you mean. That's because arthritis is a symptom, not a disease, and it has more than 100 different causes. But any joint that hurts is arthritic.

The term *arthritis* is a combination of the Greek words *arthrus* and *itis*, which, respectively, mean "joint," and "inflammation" or "infection."

Anyone can get some form of arthritis at any age. The most common types, affecting 10 percent of the population, are, in their order of frequency, osteoarthritis, rheumatoid arthritis, and gout.

The Many Faces of Arthritis

This chapter is all about osteoarthritis (OA), the type specifically associated with aging. However, before concluding that your achy joints are due to OA, consider these other possibilities:

- A fall that injures your knee gives you *traumatic arthritis.*
- A bug that infects you, enters your bloodstream, and makes its way to one or more of your joints causes *septic arthritis* (gonorrhea is one example; tuberculosis and various fungi are others).
- Your immune system can induce a *reactive arthritis* in response to various infectious agents. These include the streptococcus that causes rheumatic fever; the viruses responsible for hepatitis B, measles, German measles, the spirochete of Lyme disease, and salmonella; or bacteria present in contaminated food and water such as shigella or campylobacter.
- Too many gout crystals in the joints can give you *gouty arthritis.*
- Systemic diseases such as sickle cell anemia among African Americans, acromegaly (due to an overproduction of growth hormone by a brain tumor), abnormal cholesterol metabolism, diabetes, chronic lung

conditions, and congenital heart disease can all result in various kinds of joint disorders.

- There is a group of arthritic conditions associated with what are called autoimmune diseases, including rheumatoid arthritis, lupus, scleroderma, polyarthritis, dermatomyositis, and others. In these disorders, the body reacts to its own healthy tissues as if they were hostile invaders and tries to reject them. The result is a host of symptoms, including painful, swollen joints.

Osteoarthritis

Osteoarthritis (OA), the most common of all joint diseases in humans, affects about 16 million Americans, mostly over age forty-five, two-thirds of whom are women. There are two types of OA, primary and secondary. The latter form can occur at any age in a joint that was previously damaged by trauma or infection.

Primary osteoarthritis is associated with aging. Although present in 2 percent of persons under the age of forty-five, it usually starts in both sexes in their forties and fifties, and increases in frequency thereafter. By age sixty-five, most people have it. Interestingly, OA does not necessarily cause symptoms, but it may be detected in a routine spine X ray in someone without a complaint in the world. OA usually affects more than one joint, typically striking the hips, knees, and spinal column, as well as the farthest joints of the fingers. Unlike so many other disorders associated with aging, although OA affects more and more people as they get older, the disease itself does not necessarily become more severe. (In fact, I have often seen symptoms improve over the years, especially lower back pain.) Nor can the severity of pain usually be correlated with the degree of enlargement or deformity of the joints. However, OA can cause considerable pain in the joints of older people and limit their range of motion.

How Arthritis Develops

Primary osteoarthritis is due to wear and tear, the price you pay for having used your joints over the course of a lifetime. Here's how and why it develops. Joints consist of several different structures: bone, ligaments, muscles, tendons, and cartilage. A normal joint is flexible, with a wide range of movements. Ligaments and muscles support a healthy joint and maintain its stability. Normal cartilage inside the joint contains water; it's compressible and elastic, so that it acts like a sponge or cushion, preventing bones from rubbing against each other.

Cartilage is affected by the aging process and the biomechanical stresses of bearing weight over time. It becomes dried out and eventually splits, fragments, and is worn away; the bones within the joint now rub against each other (that hurts); they thicken, harden, and form spurs or outgrowths at the joint margins. That's basically what osteoarthritis is all about. Recent research suggests that although the wear-and-tear component is important, there may be other factors—hormonal, genetic, or immunologic—that predispose to osteoarthritis.

The erosion of cartilage is not necessarily progressive or inevitable. Early on, cartilage can regenerate and repair itself. However, as OA progresses, nature's self-maintenance and repair mechanisms become less effective; inflammatory cells move into the joint, and enzymes further break down the cartilage. When this degradation is faster than the repair process, the joint cartilage is irreversibly eroded.

Symptoms of Osteoarthritis

Osteoarthritis primarily affects the weight-bearing joints, causing pain and stiffness of the neck, back, hip, swelling of the knees, the base of the thumb, the ends of the fingers, and the big toes. These symptoms begin insidiously, usually as brief morning stiffness, progressing to increased pain with weight bearing that's relieved with rest. You feel worst first thing in the morning and improve during the day as you limber up. However, heavy activity, such as gardening, housework, or a long walk, is painful. The joints may enlarge or become deformed, but usually remain cool.

Diagnosing Osteoarthritis

Anyone with any form of arthritis should have a thorough checkup: a complete physical exam, a careful past history taken, especially with respect to previous joint injury, and an evaluation of the function of the joints in question. Pertinent blood tests, urine analysis, examination of the fluid removed from the joints, X rays (which demonstrate narrowing of the joint space, eroded cartilage, and bony overgrowth), CAT scans, MRIs, arthroscopy (direct visualization of the interior of the joint), and biopsy of joint or muscle tissue may be necessary. Always ask why a particular test is being done, how much it will cost, whether your insurance or HMO will pay for it, and how it will affect the diagnosis and treatment of your disease. There is a tendency these days to overtest patients with arthritis.

Treating Osteoarthritis

Although there is no cure for osteoarthritis, the right treatment can relieve pain and inflammation, maintain function and mobility of the joints, prevent their deformity, and enhance the quality of your life. But therapy must be tailored to your individual needs. Below are some ways to ease the pain.

Physiotherapy is a mainstay treatment for osteoarthritis. Your physiotherapist prescribes a wide range of exercises. *Isometric* and *isotonic exercise* improve muscle tone, increase flexibility, reduce stiffness, and keep you mobile; stretching increases mobility. But don't let anyone push you into doing more exercise than you're comfortable with. *Isometric* exercises contract the muscles without moving the joint; they improve muscle strength and help it support the joint. Tightening the quadriceps while sitting or standing is an example of an isometric exercise. *Isotonic* exercise adds joint movement to muscle contraction. *Aerobic exercise*—biking, swimming, and dancing—increases blood flow to the joints and strengthens the muscles surrounding them. *Weight-bearing exercise* improves joint pain and swelling, fatigue, malaise, and depression, and does not worsen arthritis.

When you're through exercising, top it all off with a delicious *massage* to relieve pain and restore movement in your joints.

You'll know you're exercising too vigorously if your pain and swelling get worse, either while you're doing it or afterwards. Never exercise a joint that's acutely inflamed, swollen, or painful. If there is any significant joint deformity or functional disability, ask for a consultation with an occupational or physical therapist before embarking on any rehabilitation program. You may need splints to reduce inflammation, to prevent contractures, and to preserve the function of the joint.

Cold packs reduce pain, inflammation, and swelling; heat relaxes muscles and stimulates their circulation. You can get that heat from a warm bath or shower, heating pad, hot packs, or an electric blanket. Some physical medicine specialists recommend alternating hot and cold compresses, starting with a hot compress for about three minutes, followed by a cold compress for thirty seconds, and repeating this procedure three times.

Here are some additional tips on maximizing the potential of your muscles and joints if you have osteoarthritis:

- Avoid keeping your muscles or joints in one position for any length of time.
- Use the strongest or largest joints for whatever task you're doing, and avoid any activity you are not able to stop immediately if you begin to hurt.
- Sit at work whenever possible.
- Don't bend, stoop, lift, or reach for items unless you absolutely must. If you have to move something, slide it if you can.
- It's easier to get off a raised toilet seat. A shower chair can make life easier for you.
- If you're doing the cooking, reduce your workload by making more than you need and freezing the rest.
- Prepare food for the coming week on the weekends, when the entire family can help.
- Use more frozen or packaged foods.
- Use lightweight utensils in the kitchen.
- Adapt the handles on cupboards and drawers, and use faucet grips and drawer openers.
- Have plenty of jar openers around and use a long-handled reacher for getting things down from high places.
- Don't be shy. Ask for help with shopping and cleaning, especially during flare-ups.

- If your fingers are arthritic, avoid shoes with laces; buy slip-ons or those with Velcro.
- Wear good shoes, use shoe inserts and a walking stick if you need them (avoid the word *cane*, it carries the same stigma as *hearing aid*). Heed your pain; it's your body's message that you're doing too much.

MEDICATIONS FOR OSTEOARTHRITIS

None of the drugs currently used to treat osteoarthritis alter its course or prevent joint destruction. If you need medication to ease your pain, use the weakest ones first. Work your way up to three or four adult aspirin or a gram of acetaminophen (Tylenol) a day. You can apply methyl salicylate or capsaicin cream to the painful joints, but these are not very potent painkillers. If Tylenol doesn't work, move on to the nonsteroidal agents (NSAIDs, such as Aleve, Advil, and Nuprin). These are good analgesics (pain reducers) and anti-inflammatory drugs, and are available without a prescription. Always take them with food and report any digestive problems or ulcer pain to your doctor. The NSAIDs may cause ulcers or erosion of the lining of the stomach and upper intestinal tract and can lead to bleeding, especially in older persons. When that happens, discontinue the drug. If the symptoms were mild, you may either resume the drug at a lower dose after a few days or switch to a different brand. To avoid these problems, if you're taking NSAIDs on an ongoing basis, I suggest you combine them with H-2 blockers (marketed as Tagamet, Axid, Zantac, Prevacid, and Prilosec). These cut down acid production in the stomach. You can also use sucralfate, which coats the stomach, or the prostaglandin analog called misoprostol, which protects the lining of the stomach from the erosion caused by NSAIDs. It reduces the incidence of NSAID-induced stomach and duodenal ulcers by about 40 percent. You can now buy it combined with an NSAID; it is marketed as diclofenac.

Chronic use of NSAIDs can also cause other complications: kidney problems, as well as liver and neurologic toxicity. But a new type has recently been released. It belongs to a group of drugs in the Cox 2 inhibitor family. They differ from conventional NSAIDs in that they control pain and inflammation without harming the stomach lining. The first of these agents is called Celebrex. The dosage is 100 milligrams a day.

If acetaminophen and NSAIDs aren't effective, stay away from habit-forming narcotics as long as you can. Arthritis is a chronic disorder, and it doesn't take much to become dependent on painkillers.

Another alternative is steroid injection into the arthritic joint. This often provides relief, but it should never be done when the joint is infected or unstable. Even though this technique does reduce pain, I do not advise more than three or four injections a year because they can damage the joint cartilage. If you need more, you should consider surgery. Long-term oral steroids are fraught with potential side effects.

Doxycycline, a member of the tetracycline family,

which is widely used to treat a variety of infections and skin conditions, may slow the progression of osteoarthritis and even prevent it. It probably works by blocking the action of the enzymes that break down joint cartilage. There is currently an ongoing study to test its effectiveness sponsored by the NIH.

"THE ARTHRITIS CURE"

The title of a best-selling book a few years ago, "The Arthritis Cure" is a misnomer. The authors state that glucosamine and chondroitin sulfate have a dramatic impact on the course of osteoarthritis. I have not found this to be so. This product does help some people with mild OA and you should try it, by all means. But don't expect a cure.

Here is how the combination of glucosamine and chondroitin is believed to work. The basic constituent of cartilage is collagen, which is woven around strands of sugar-carrying proteins called proteoglycans. These proteoglycans, a combination of chondroitin and keratin sulfate, trap molecules of water to give the cartilage its cushioning properties. As we get older, cartilage cells make fewer proteoglycans, resulting in a breakdown of the cartilage. Presumably, taking chondroitin sulfate, which is a type of proteoglycan, can help restore the cushioning properties of the cartilage.

Glucosamine is a building block of mucopolysaccharides, which are compounds normally present in the membranes, ligaments, tendons, and cartilage that make up the joints and the fluid that bathes and lubricates them. A deficiency of glucosamine leaves the synovial fluid thin and watery, and less able to lubricate and cushion the moving parts in the joint. Glucosamine supplements are said by their proponents to thicken this fluid.

There have been several reports in the European literature attesting to the efficacy of glucosamine. I have not seen any reports of toxicity.

SURGERY FOR OSTEOARTHRITIS

When osteoarthritis is severe and crippling, and affects the quality of your life, several joints such as the shoulder, knee, and hip can be replaced by prostheses made of a combination of metal or plastic. These operations are more than 90 percent successful. However, there are several other less drastic and invasive procedures to consider first.

Arthroscopy, the introduction of a diagnostic/therapeutic instrument, permits the doctor to perform a synovectomy, in which the (synovial) tissue lining the joint is removed. This can slow the progression of disease and substantially reduce pain. Unfortunately, symptoms often recur, so synovectomy is of limited usefulness over the long term.

The joint can be repaired by an invasive operative procedure called *arthroplasty*. When successful, its effects last for about ten or fifteen years. It's worth looking into.

If these less complicated procedures aren't successful, the arthritic joint can be replaced. It's very important for you to know that artificial joints are prone to infection from bacteria released into the bloodstream during tooth cleaning, extractions, root canals, or other dental surgery. It's very much like having a diseased or artificial heart valve. You must take prophylactic antibiotics before having *any* dental work. This is especially true if you have diabetes, rheumatoid arthritis, or are taking steroids or other immune-suppressing drugs that leave you vulnerable to infection.

Medication Problems

There are many potential problems associated with the medical treatment of arthritis, especially in the elderly. They may take the wrong dose of their medication; the drugs can have adverse reactions or interact with other medications (especially blood thinners) and with food; and treatment can interfere with laboratory tests. Although Tylenol has none of the gastrointestinal hazards of the NSAIDs, it also has no anti-inflammatory effect, and so doesn't usually provide adequate relief. The salicylates are inexpensive but can be toxic. Combining diclofenac and misoprostol costs about $132 a month, and can cause diarrhea. One-third or more of acute intestinal bleeds from NSAIDs in the elderly occur without warning. If you're taking any of these drugs, you must have a regular hemoglobin test and an examination of your stool for blood, which may not be apparent to the naked eye. Combining aspirin and NSAIDs substantially increases the risk of such a bleed.

TREATING OSTEOARTHRITIS OF THE KNEE

Osteoarthritis of the knee is the leading cause of disability among the elderly and deserves special mention here. It's twice as common in women—approximately 2 percent of elderly females develop it—and it's usually more severe than in men.

The knee is a complex joint; it connects the two longest bones in the body, the shinbone (tibia) and the thighbone (femur). It normally has a wide range of motion and is extremely important in helping to support the weight of the body. There is a recent development in the management of osteoarthritis of the knee of which you should be aware. To understand how it works, we need first to review what happens when osteoarthritis strikes the knee.

Remember that the space between the bones in the knee joint contains synovial fluid that acts as a cushion between them. When osteoarthritis develops, this fluid becomes thin and is a less effective shock absorber. This further exposes the cartilage, which is now more vulnerable to impact and friction. Your knee hurts when you bear weight because of the increased sensitivity of the nerve endings in the soft tissues of the joint. As the disease progresses, the unprotected cartilage begins to wear away, becomes less smooth, and breaks down. The bones, normally protected by the cartilage and the synovial fluid, harden and form bone spurs that rub against each other. Even the most minor movement of the knee is painful.

The new therapy for the knee consists of the injection of a substance into the synovial space in the knee joint to enhance the elasticity and thickness of the synovial fluid. This material is a solution of hyaluronate, a component of healthy synovial fluid that occurs naturally in the knee joint. It is marketed in the United States as Hyalgan and Synvisc. When injected directly into the knee, hyaluronate is said to reduce pain and leave the joint more supple and flexible. A course of treatment usually consists of one injection a week for four or five weeks. You should rest the knee for about forty-eight hours after the injection. This treatment should never be done if your knee joint is infected or if you're pregnant or nursing. The only side effects reported so far are occasional temporary, localized discomfort, and itching, a rash, or swelling at the site of injection. Since hyaluronate comes from rooster combs, you may not be able to tolerate it if you're allergic to feathers, eggs, or poultry. The benefits from one course of treatment usually last about six months and sometimes longer. If you have osteoarthritis of the knee, discuss hyaluronate treatment with your doctor, but don't expect miracles. The drug is expensive and few of my own patients who have tried it so far have given it rave reviews. However, it has helped some.

EXERCISE AND OSTEOARTHRITIS

Normal exercise and day-to-day living do not cause or accelerate degenerative joint disease. A moderate regular exercise program is good for you at any age if you haven't had any previous joint problems. Your joints are living structures; their cells are continually renewing themselves and adapting to the load you place on them. The more you use them, the better off you are. Remember, however, that previous injury to a joint does leave it more vulnerable to osteoarthritis.

If you're middle-aged or older and have begun to develop osteoarthritis but want to engage in some sport or exercise, there's no reason not to do so.

What kind of exercise should you do? Low-impact activities such as recreational swimming, golf, ballroom dancing, and walking can all improve strength and mobility in older people, even those with mild to moderate osteoarthritis. If your muscles are healthy and your joints are normal, you may safely engage in moderate-level activities such as bowling, bicycling, or rowing. However, avoid high-risk sports such as baseball, softball, and basketball, because when a joint is subjected to a stress or force, the cartilage fluid distributes the impact evenly. When that force or movement is sudden or repetitive, as in jumping or running, or when there is a twisting motion, the joint cartilage and muscles may not have time to absorb the shock properly. This increases the likelihood of its injury. That's why so many football, baseball, and soccer players and other athletes are at high risk for damaging their joints.

DIET AND OSTEOARTHRITIS

The most important role of diet in the prevention or treatment of osteoarthritis is weight loss, even if joint destruction is already advanced. You can do this most effectively by adhering to a low-fat, low-calorie diet and exercising regularly. Weight loss relieves joint pain by decreasing the stress on the joints and the destruction within them. One hears a great deal about the allergic component of arthritis, but I have never seen any evidence of it, as far as osteoarthritis is concerned. Although it makes sense to eliminate any food that appears to worsen your condition, don't waste a whole lot of time trying to figure it out.

ALTERNATIVE MEDICINE FOR OSTEOARTHRITIS

Practitioners of alternative medicine would disagree with my rather negative comments about the role of diet in the causation of osteoarthritis. Some claim that since vitamins A, C, B_6, as well as copper and zinc, are all required to make collagen and cartilage, the following supplements should be taken daily both to prevent and to treat osteoarthritis: 10,000 units of vitamin A; 2,000 to 3,000 units of vitamin C; 600 units of vitamin E; 50 milligrams of vitamin B_6; 45 milligrams of zinc; 1 milligram of copper; 12 1/2 milligrams of pantothenic acid; and 250 milligrams of methionine, an amino acid said to be important in maintaining healthy cartilage. I have seen no studies showing that the administration of this formula makes any difference. It's a purely theoretical concept. If you can afford to buy these items, there's probably no downside to taking them.

Acupuncture is another alternative-therapy option. I routinely prescribe it as part of any physiotherapy program.

Naturopaths and others also recommend the use of various herbal remedies to help osteoarthritis. These include tincture of yucca leaf, tea containing devil's claw, and alfalfa-leaf extract. Again, I know of no scientific evidence that these herbs work.

What to Remember about Osteoarthritis

1. Osteoarthritis is the form of arthritis specifically related to aging.
2. Arthritis is a symptom, not a disease. There are more than 100 different causes of joint pain.
3. Osteoarthritis is not necessarily progressive, and symptoms sometimes improve with age.
4. Osteoarthritis results from the breakdown of cartilage and the hardening and thickening of the bones of the joints.
5. The major cause of osteoarthritis is believed to be long-term wear and tear, but genetic, immunologic, and hormonal factors may also play a role.

6. The basic treatment of osteoarthritis is a combination of physiotherapy, a balance between rest and exercise, weight loss, pain medication, and various surgical procedures, including joint replacement.

7. There are no medications that cure osteoarthritis, but they can provide effective pain relief. Be aware that aspirin and the nonsteroidal anti-inflammatory drugs can cause bleeding from the upper gastrointestinal tract.

12

OSTEOPOROSIS

Hip, Hip, Hooray

When you're young and healthy, a hefty sneeze will generate no more than a "God bless you" from a well-wisher; a hacking cough left over from a bad cold may cause some dirty looks from those sitting near you in the theater; if you slip or trip and fall, chances are you'll just scrape your knees or twist an ankle. But if you're a woman beyond your fifties or sixties and your periods are just a memory, a vigorous sneeze or cough may break one of your ribs, and a trivial fall may well result in a fractured hip or some other broken bone. Your body responds differently at age twenty-five than when you're seventy because the drop in estrogen production that begins at menopause causes your bones to lose some of their calcium, to become thinner and brittle, and to break more easily. That's osteoporosis.

Osteoporosis: The Problem

Women don't worry much about osteoporosis when they're young. The threat is years away, and not nearly as emotionally devastating as the prospect of Alzheimer's, a massive stroke, a serious heart attack, or cancer. Yet osteoporosis can have very dire consequences, and it is more common than most of the other trappings of aging. For example, it's bad enough that one woman in eight will develop breast cancer in her lifetime, but if you're female and over fifty, there's a 50 percent chance that you will one day break a bone! Twenty-eight million women in this country (and a forgotten cohort of almost 5 million men, many of whom have an alcohol problem or low levels of the male hormone, testosterone) sustain about 1 1/2 million fractures every year. When you're young, that amounts to nothing more than a plaster cast for a week or two; a nuisance, but no big deal. However, 60,000 of the 300,000 persons who break a hip every year die during the twelve months after their accident, usually from such complications of prolonged bed rest as pneumonia or embolism (a traveling blood clot) to the lungs. Among the 240,000 "lucky" enough to survive the fracture itself, one in four ends up in a nursing home within a year, no longer able to care for herself.

Even if it doesn't result in an obvious bone break, osteoporosis takes its toll in other ways. Calcium gradually and insidiously seeps out of the bones of the spine, causing them to develop "micro" fractures and ultimately to collapse. The result is chronic back pain, loss of height, and deformity of the spine (the familiar "dowager's hump").

The irony of it all is that the best time to prevent osteoporosis is when it's the farthest thing from your mind. For prevention to be most effective, you've got to start it early in life and never let up.

Even if you already have some evidence of osteoporosis (usually because you waited too long to begin preventive measures), you can still halt its progress and even reverse some of the damage it has already caused.

How and Why Osteoporosis Happens

Unlike all those skeletons in the museum, or the bones of dead animals strewn in farm fields, your bones are alive; they're as vibrant and as dynamic as any other organ in the body, and they respond to physical stress in much the same way. Their blood vessels deliver and remove calcium, other nutrients, and hormones.

Bone consists of a protein framework wrapped in calcium. Its strength and "breakability" depend on its calcium content—the more, the better. Throughout life, there is a constant process of absorption and resorption of calcium in living bone. This is carried out by two kinds of cells: osteoblasts that add calcium and osteoclasts that remove it. These cells, in turn, respond to a wide variety of changes in the body's internal environment. The net amount of calcium present in your bones when you begin menopause depends on the proper balance between osteoblastic and osteoclastic activity over the years, and how much of this mineral was laid down in your bones when you were young.

The calcium in your diet is absorbed from the intestinal tract; 90 percent of it ends up in your bones and teeth. But calcium also moves in the other direction—it's sucked *out* of bone, too. Which process predominates, the "in" or the "out," depends on your age, hormonal status, the needs of your bones, the stress to which they're subjected, and how much calcium is required by competing biological processes such as muscle contraction and blood clotting.

When you're young, your bones acquire more calcium than they lose. Between thirty and forty years of age, the process equalizes so that the same amount is deposited as lost. At or about menopause, the osteoclasts begin to take over, and more calcium is removed than laid down. This happens for two main reasons: There is less estrogen produced by the ovaries at this time of life (remember, it's estrogen that stops calcium loss). Also, as we grow older, our gut absorbs less of the calcium we eat, and so there's not as much available for deposit on the bones.

Most calcium is lost from bone at two stages in a woman's life—first, soon after her periods end, and then some fifteen years later. This "negative calcium balance," if continued unchecked, leads to the thin bones of osteoporosis.

Are *You* at Risk for Osteoporosis?

Whether or not your bones become osteoporotic depends mainly on how much calcium was deposited on them when you were young, and also how much estrogen your body was making during those formative years. But there are other important determinants. Some, like genetic makeup, are beyond our control, but we can do something about several of the others. Following are the major risk factors for osteoporosis.

• **Your family history:** If your mother, sister, or grandmother fractured her bones, especially the hip, you're at twice the risk for a similar fate.

• **Caucasian and Asian women** are more vulnerable to osteoporosis than are Afro-Americans. Females with a *fair complexion, light-colored hair,* and a *small body frame* are also more likely to develop it. I haven't seen many overweight ladies with thin bones. Obesity (which has several other disadvantages) is actually associated with less osteoporosis, presumably because extra weight stresses the bones, which then call for and receive more calcium. Fat cells may also store estrogen.

• **A sedentary lifestyle:** Just sitting around, without making demands on your bones, reduces their need for calcium. Later in life, when what little calcium you did lay down begins to seep out, you're in trouble.

• **You need to consume enough calcium over the years.** It's very much like money in the bank: If you save while you're working, it's available when you re-tire. If you avoided calcium in your diet because you thought that the dairy products that contain it would make you fat, or you are lactose intolerant and milk makes you sick, or you wanted to lower your choles-terol—and despite the poor dietary intake, you didn't add calcium supplements to your diet—you're a good candidate for osteoporosis.

• **If you had a trivial injury and ended up with a surprise fracture,** chances are your bones aren't as solid as they should be. Get yourself tested (see below) to determine their actual calcium content.

• **If you've been taking steroid hormones** (cortisonelike drugs) for more than six months for any reason (arthritis, asthma, cancer, or to prevent rejection after receiving an organ transplant), you're at substantial risk for osteoporosis. These hormones leave the bones with too little calcium because they reduce the amount that is absorbed by the gut. Also, calcium circulating in the bloodstream is normally reabsorbed by the kidney and not excreted in the urine. It's too precious to pee away. These steroids block the reabsorption process so that calcium is lost in the urine. Finally, they increase the activity of the osteoclasts that suck out what calcium there is in bone. So when you're taking steroid hormones for any length of time, your bones are getting a triple whammy, the net result of which is osteoporosis.

Other medications such as the anti-epilepsy drugs phenobarbital, primidone, and phenytoin, as well as thyroid hormone, have a similar but not nearly as powerful a thinning effect on bone as steroids. Women with epilepsy should discuss with their doctors the use of one of the other newer agents for this disorder. If you have a sluggish thyroid gland, make sure that you're not getting more replacement thyroid hormone than you need. Excess may lead to abnormally thin bones. If you have an overactive thyroid (hyperthyroidism), it's the same as taking too much replacement hormone for an underfunctioning gland. No matter where it comes from, too much thyroid hormone leads to osteoporosis.

• **If a substantial part of your stomach** or intestinal tract was surgically removed, there is now a smaller area from which dietary calcium can be absorbed. This leaves less calcium available for deposit in your bones.

• **The parathyroid glands** are tiny structures located above the thyroid gland in the neck. They cannot be seen or felt, even when they're enlarged. They make a hormone that controls the flow of calcium in and out of the bones. When the parathyroid gland makes too much of this hormone (hyperparathyroidism), either because it's overactive or it contains a tumor, calcium is sucked out of the bones, leaving them brittle and osteoporotic.

• **Other less common causes** of calcium loss are kidney diseases that result in the excretion of abnormally large amounts of calcium, and certain malignancies such as multiple myeloma, lymphoma, and leukemia.

• **If you're a smoker,** you'll have 5 to 50 percent less calcium in your bones by the time menopause rolls around. That's because tobacco interferes with the protective effects of estrogen on bone.

• **If you had less than normal exposure to estrogen** throughout your life, you are a candidate for osteoporosis. This can happen in several different ways: You may be estrogen-deficient because both ovaries were removed for some reason and you did not receive adequate estrogen replacement therapy (ERT). (A simple hysterectomy, in which the uterus was removed but the ovaries were left in place, doesn't count because the uterus does not make estrogen.) You may have hypogonadism—failure of your sex organs to develop properly so that they do not make enough estrogen. Perhaps your periods didn't start until you were sixteen or older, or your menopause had its onset much earlier than normal (in your thirties or early forties rather than sometime near fifty). Or maybe you were a vigorous athlete and frequently missed your periods for six months or longer. The price you pay for being "fit" is the loss of much of your body fat, and decreased storage and production of estrogen. All these conditions leave you with less estrogen over the years and a possible calcium deficiency in your bones.

• **If you were confined to bed for six months or longer,** especially when you were an adolescent, you may have lost enough bone mass to make you osteoporotic later on.

• **If you have a history of chronic alcohol excess,** your calcium absorption from the gut is probably less than normal. Alcohol also reduces the positive effect of estrogen on bone. So restrict your daily intake of booze to five ounces of wine, or a half-ounce of liquor, or twelve ounces of beer.

• **I generally advise my female patients to limit their coffee intake to three cups a day** because high caffeine intake increases the amount of calcium passed in the urine. I advise them to drink at least one glass of milk to counter the negative effect caffeine has on bone. However, you coffee lovers will be glad to know that more recent studies conducted at the University of Pennsylvania have failed to confirm this link between coffee consumption and osteoporosis. Let's wait and see who's right.

• **Bone density in women who were depressed was re-cently found to be 6.5 percent lower** than it is in their happier counterparts. That may be because higher blood levels of cortisol, a stress hormone that predisposes to osteoporosis, often accompany depression. So if you're depressed, here's what to do: Get your bone density tested, review your life situation and take the necessary steps to improve your mood, make sure you're getting enough calcium in your diet, engage regularly in weight-bearing exercise, and ask your doctor about taking hormonal supplements.

How to Prevent Osteoporosis

Now that you know the major risk factors for osteoporosis and their effects, try to modify them. Let's consider them one by one:

• **Family history:** Forget about having any impact on this one. I'm afraid you're stuck with your parents and your siblings. We may someday be able to alter our genetic patterns, but not yet.

• **If you're Caucasian or Asian and female:** There's nothing you can do about your race. Ditto for your sex. If you're female, forget about a sex change; it really isn't worth it. And for men, taking estrogen will give you larger breasts, less facial hair, and zero sex drive, but it won't make your bones any stronger! Some doctors are prescribing two nonhormonal agents for men who either have osteoporosis or are prone to it. Calcitonin (Miacalcin) and alendronate (Fosamax), discussed below, may be beneficial, but there haven't been enough studies to show that they are effective.

- **Fair complexion, light-colored hair, and small body frame:** That's something else you're stuck with. Tanning your skin and dyeing your hair won't make a difference. Neither will high heels.

- **A sedentary lifestyle:** Now you're talking! Weight-bearing exercises throughout life, ideally started by age twenty-five and done regularly, are probably the most effective way to prevent osteoporosis. Get into the habit of walking for forty-five to sixty minutes at least three or four times a week. The days you're not walking, lift weights for thirty minutes. Jogging and dancing are good, too. My son, Arthur, the tai chi teacher, is convinced, as are many osteoporosis specialists, that these oriental exercises prevent falls in the elderly by improving their balance. Swimming, on the other hand, does not involve bearing weight, and although it's great for muscles and joints, it doesn't do much for bones and won't prevent osteoporosis.

- **Enough calcium in the diet:** I'm not convinced by the results of a Harvard study that concluded that adequate dietary calcium throughout your life does not help prevent osteoporosis after menopause. Make calcium a staple part of your diet virtually from day one. The 400 to 600 milligrams of calcium that the average American consumes daily is not enough. You need at least 1,200 milligrams during adolescence and 1,500 milligrams after menopause (unless you're taking estrogen replacement, in which case 1,000 milligrams a day will do). You should be able to get these amounts from your diet unless you avoid dairy products such as milk and cheese (which many people do because they're worried about their cholesterol or their weight). In that case, drink skim milk or eat nonfat yogurt or low-fat cheese. They contain negligible amounts of cholesterol. If, for any reason, you're not getting enough calcium in your food, then take supplements. I recommend calcium carbonate and calcium citrate. The carbonate is cheaper than the citrate and provides 40 percent elemental calcium in each tablet, as compared to only 24 percent from the citrate. Have them with food for maximum absorption. Although ERT after menopause is the single most important factor in preventing osteoporosis, you can slow its progress for at least three to six years by taking adequate amounts of calcium *after* menopause.

• **You need at least 400 units of vitamin D every day** (some doctors prescribe 800 units) to keep your bones strong. This vitamin promotes the absorption of calcium by the gut and into the bones. Its richest natural source is the action of sunlight on the skin. If you don't spend enough time outdoors because you're homebound, or live in Scandinavia where there is no sun for many months a year, then drink four or five glasses of skim milk fortified with vitamin D daily. Unlike the water-soluble vitamins such as vitamin C, of which any excess you take is excreted in the urine, too much vitamin D can be harmful. If you're not sure about your vitamin D levels, there's a simple blood test that will provide the answer.

• **Soybeans and other plant compounds** contain phytoestrogens, many of whose actions mimic those of estrogen. Soy protein comes in a powder that can be conveniently added to juice, sodas, or baked into bread. It also improves cholesterol levels and minimizes the hot flashes of menopause.

• **If you're taking any medication that can cause osteoporosis** (steroid hormones, certain anti-epilepsy drugs, too much thyroid replacement), you and your doctor should either consider some other therapy or modify the dosage. However, there has been a breakthrough as far as steroids and osteoporosis are concerned. Bone loss caused by steroids can be prevented by intermittent therapy with etidronate (Didronel), a drug used in the treatment of osteoporosis (see below). The recommended regimen consists of four cycles, each of 400 milligrams of etidronate a day for fourteen days, followed by 500 milligrams of calcium daily for the next seventy-six days. Steroid hormones have the same adverse effect on men's bones as they do on women's bones. What's more, they also reduce the amount of testosterone circulating in the body, further decreasing the calcium supply to the bones. According to recent studies, supplemental male hormone (testosterone) will significantly protect men against the ravages of steroid-induced osteoporosis.

• **Stop smoking—now.** It's never too late. Not only will your bones remain stronger longer, you'll reap many other benefits too. You'll have more money in your pocket, less cancer in your body, and a stronger heart.

• **Women! Don't go through life with a low estrogen level.** Take estrogen replacement therapy if you've had *both* ovaries removed. If one ovary or any portion of it was spared, you're getting enough estrogen. Also, if you're a professional athlete and usually miss your periods, chances are you have too little estrogen around to protect your bones. You may need to be hormonally "touched up" during your athletic career.

Replacing the missing estrogen at menopause is the single most important thing you can do to minimize or prevent your bones from losing their calcium. We've known for many years that estrogen prevents the hot flashes that often accompany menopause. Nor is it a secret that women who use it look younger, feel better, and have a longer and better sex life. But that's only the tip of the iceberg. Estrogen also protects against osteoporosis, heart disease, stroke, and Alzheimer's. Still, it may not be right for you if you have breast cancer or some other malignancy, migraines, liver or gallbladder problems, high blood pressure, abnormal blood fats, especially high triglycerides (neutral fat), or a history of blood clots. So you and your doctor should weigh the pros and cons in your particular case and decide together whether hormone replacement therapy is for you. Remember too that despite its many major benefits, there are potential risks and side effects to ERT. I understand that two of every three women who start ERT discontinue it after two years. That's largely because they fear breast cancer. If you have a strong family history of this malignancy, you probably shouldn't take estrogen. Another downside to ERT is the fact that your menstrual cycles may resume after you've started it (unless, of course, you've had a hysterectomy). Even the symptoms of PMS that tormented you during your fertile years—the depression, breast soreness, mood changes, headaches, and fluid retention—may return. Endometriosis (one of nature's mistakes in which uterine tissue lining makes its way to other organs such as the ovaries, pelvic wall, or fallopian tubes) may flare up after you start taking estrogen. This may mean a return of the pain you used to have with your periods before your menopause. These fears and side effects should all be addressed before you make a final decision about ERT.

• **If you're vulnerable to osteoporosis for any of the reasons mentioned above, limit your alcohol intake** to the amounts I suggested earlier. There's much to be said for the health-promoting properties of booze in moderate quantities, but it has a negative effect if you cross the line.

• **You're also better off avoiding excessive salt,** which some doctors think leaches calcium from bone.

Detecting Osteoporosis *before* Your Bones Break

Now that you know the risk factors for osteoporosis and how to prevent them, how can you tell whether or not you've been successful in your efforts? If your bones have continued to leak calcium and are getting thinner and thinner despite the preventive measures you've taken, there are several treatment options. So don't wait for the first break, or for the bones in your spine to "melt" away, before evaluating the status of your skeletal system. The best way to do that is by densitometry, in which an X-ray beam is narrowly focused on some combination of bones such as the hip, spine, wrist, and occasionally the whole body. Make sure that at least two bones are studied, the hip and one other. Densitometry is quick, painless, and the newer techniques expose you to very little radiation. Every menopausal woman and anyone else who is vulnerable to osteoporosis should have it done. Unlike mammography, there are as yet no official guidelines as to when to do so. And unfortunately, you'll probably have to ask for it yourself, because at last count, two-thirds of the primary care doctors in the United States (who should know better) don't tell their patients about it! Medicare is currently paying between $100 and $120 for densitometry, but their reimbursements change so often I suggest you check it out before you have your test. Half the private insurers I contacted do not cover densitometry at all.

Have your densitometry done at a center that performs lots of it. Chances are the results will be interpreted more accurately at such a facility. Avoid "storefront" clinics that advertise. Also, ask for the dual energy X-ray absorptiometry (DXA or DEXA) technique. It's the latest method that uses a double beam of low-intensity X rays; it takes less than fifteen minutes to do and exposes you to no more radiation than what you'd get on a transcontinental flight.

If you can't find a facility with DXA equipment near you (there are currently fewer than 1,000 in the United States), some of the other techniques are acceptable. They produce somewhat more radiation, but still very little. These include dual photon absorptiometry; quantitative computed tomography (QTC) to study the bones of the spine; peripheral QTC to examine the wrists; radiographic absorptiometry for the hands; and several others. If your own doctor doesn't have the information you need, you can obtain a list of the approved densitometry centers in your area by calling the National Osteoporosis Foundation at 1-800-464-6700.

Densitometry results are not absolute. They compare how your bones stack up against those of someone much younger, say twenty-five or thirty years of age. It's no use pitting your pictures against those of a woman your own age because you may both have osteoporosis.

There is currently ongoing research to develop ultrasound as a less expensive, radiation-free way to detect osteoporosis. This would measure the vibration of bone responding to sound waves directed to it. Fascinating idea, but still a ways off.

Common Sense Measures if You Have Osteoporosis

In addition to the available treatments for osteoporosis that slow down or stop the loss of calcium from your bones, and even restore it, there are some other practical, common-sense measures to follow. Their main goal is to keep you from *falling*.

Avoid medications that make you drowsy or impair your balance. The greatest offenders are sedatives, antidepressants, anti-anxiety agents, and antihistamines. If you must take them, stay put—and seated—until their effects wear off. Prolonged exposure to cold can also leave you less alert by lowering your body temperature.

Get rid of slippery throw rugs. Give them to your kids whose bones can withstand a fall; remove loose extension cords (both my mother and my mother-in-law fell in *my* home and fractured their knees because of this); don't leave any of your grandchildren's toys lying around after they've gone home; pick up after your dog, too—many a human bone has been broken falling over a canine's. Equip your home, especially your bathroom and bathtub, with nonskid mats; put grab bars in your tub and near your toilet; install handrails on all staircases as well as by your swimming pool; and make sure your home is adequately lit.

Here are some other personal measures you should take: Avoid high heels; you're better off with rubber-soled shoes, more of which are becoming available in fashionable styles. Don't change position suddenly—as we get older, our arteries become more rigid and don't adjust to blood pressure changes as promptly as when we were young. When you stand up quickly after you've been lying down or sitting, you may become dizzy and fall. Finally, check your vision regularly.

If you do fracture a bone, ask for whatever painkillers are necessary to control your pain, get into a good physiotherapy program, and don't be shy about using any appliances and/or braces that can support the fractured bone until it heals. You want to avoid lots of "rest," which will thin your bones even further.

Treating Osteoporosis before and after the Fractures

The prevention and treatment of osteoporosis are a continuum. After the diagnosis is made (by densitometry, or because you've shrunk or broken a bone after a minor injury), keep doing everything you did to prevent it in the first place. Regular weight-bearing exercises, enough calcium in your diet or calcium supplements, and estrogen replacement therapy are all now more important than ever. Make no bones about that! Estrogen not only slows down the process of demineralization, it can help restore some of what was lost. So continue to take it, by all means.

You're less likely to have side effects from ERT if you take the right amount tailored to your body's needs. That should be at least 0.625 milligrams of oral estrogen daily. Anything less than that is not likely to prevent osteoporosis. Note that estrogen therapy alone doubles the risk of cancer of the uterus. However, adding another female hormone, progestin, eliminates that risk. You can take an estrogen-progestin combination together all month, or you can do it cyclically. The continuous replacement daily regimen consists of 2.5 to 5 milligrams of progestin and 0.625 milligrams of estrogen. The usual cyclic method involves daily doses of estrogen for twenty-one days a month, and oral progestin for the last ten to fourteen days of the cycle. I suggest you opt for fourteen days because recent studies suggest that anything less than that leaves you at increased risk for uterine cancer. Cyclic hormonal replacement therapy causes menstrual-like bleeding. The continuous combined therapy using lower doses of progestin is just as effective as the cyclical regimen with the higher daily amounts.

If ERT gives you unpleasant or intolerable side effects, try a smaller dose before abandoning it (but no less than the 0.625 milligrams). If that doesn't work for you, switch to the estrogen patch. It can be applied anywhere on the abdomen, and it releases the estrogen directly through the skin. Topical estrogen doesn't get to the liver like it does when you take it by mouth. So this is the preferred method if you have liver or gallbladder disease, or clotting problems (since the liver makes the clotting factors in the blood). You're also less likely to have migraines from the patch, since its estrogen circulates throughout the body with fewer fluctuations in level.

Some doctors also claim success against osteoporosis with vaginal rings containing estradiol, a form of estrogen. Side effects are said to be minimal.

A word of caution: There is a new and exciting antidiabetic drug called troglitazone (marketed as Rezulin), which increases sensitivity to insulin. This means that it can reduce the amount of insulin required, or even eliminate its need in some adult diabetics. Rezulin also enhances the breakdown of estrogen in the liver, leaving less of the hormone available to your body's tissues. Such lower estrogen levels may reduce its effectiveness against osteoporosis. So if you're taking Rezulin for your diabetes, ask your doctor whether you should have more estrogen. (If you're younger and using the pill for contraception, Rezulin may similarly reduce its hormone content and efficacy. Be sure to discuss this with your doctor too.)

If you can't or won't take estrogen, there are other bone-protecting measures available. Some have been around for a while; others are recent. the most important one is *alendronate* (marketed in the United States as *Fosamax.*) It's not a hormone, and so doesn't have any of the other benefits of estrogen, such as lowering the risk of vascular disease and Alzheimer's. But neither does it cause breast or uterine cancer. Fosamax works by blocking the resorption of calcium that occurs after menopause and allows normal bone formation to continue. It is as effective as estrogen in preventing bone fractures, it works faster than estrogen, and its benefits may continue for longer. The usual dose is 10 milligrams a day, but you must be careful to take it in a very special way: first thing in the morning with six to eight ounces of water. Eat nothing for the next half-hour, and don't lie down. Unless you follow these instructions to the letter, you'll irritate your foodpipe and experience troublesome "indigestion." Fosamax is safe and effective, and has been shown to reduce the incidence of fractures throughout the body. Some doctors are combining it with estrogen for maximal effect. If you continue to experience chest pain, heartburn, or pain on swallowing despite using it as directed, tell your doctor.

Calcitonin is another effective anti-osteoporosis drug. It's an amino-acid polypeptide made by the thyroid gland, and it works by decreasing the activity of the osteoclasts, the calcium suckers (as opposed to the osteoblasts, which lay calcium down). Calcitonin used to be available only by injection, in which form it caused nausea and other side effects. But it now comes in a nasal spray (marketed in the United States as *Miacalcin*) without any of these side effects. You squirt it into one nostril every day. Calcitonin has the additional beneficial effect of being a mild painkiller, so if you've already had a bone break due to your osteoporosis, Miacalcin will not only help prevent another one, it will make you more comfortable, too. Although Miacalcin is a useful agent, it's not quite as effective as Fosamax.

Etidronate (marketed as *Didronel* in the United States) is an oral preparation, which, like calcitonin, reduces bone resorption by interfering with the activity of the osteoclasts. It's taken on an empty stomach two hours after eating, and you should not have any food for the next two hours. Most patients prefer to take it at bedtime. The therapy is cyclical—two weeks every three months. This is the drug you should be taking if you are receiving long-term steroid therapy. It has been shown to help prevent osteoporosis caused by the cortisone family of drugs.

The hottest medication on the market against osteoporosis is *raloxifene (Evista)*. This drug has both estrogen-potentiating and anti-estrogen properties. On the one hand it prevents bone loss just as estrogen does, but on the other, it has also been shown to lower the risk of breast cancer by as much as 75 percent. These findings came on the heels of the news that tamoxifen, a drug used in the treatment of breast cancer, lowers the risk by 44 percent. (I didn't believe Dr. Larry Norton, a cancer specialist at the Sloan-Kettering Memorial Hospital, when he predicted recently that cancer of the breast would be a thing of the past in our lifetime. Given all these new data, he may be right!)

There is also an extremely promising medication not yet available in the United States at the time of writing. But ask your doctor about it because by the time this book is published, the FDA may have approved it. I'm referring to sodium fluoride, the stuff we add to drinking water to prevent our kids from having dental cavities. Because it worked so well for that, someone came up with the idea that it might also protect bones from osteoporosis. So for several years, thousands of women were given sodium fluoride as a test. Unfortunately, the results were not impressive. In fact, despite the observation that fluoride actually makes more bone-forming osteoblasts, it sometimes worsened osteoporosis. However, recent studies have shown that the long-acting form of fluoride does improve osteoporosis. Keep an eye open for it.

What to Remember about Osteoporosis

1. Sticks and stones may not break your bones if you understand what causes osteoporosis and understand that this common, deadly complication of aging can be avoided.
2. Calcium is lost from the bones at menopause because of a decreased level of the female hormone, estrogen. This leaves them thin, brittle, and vulnerable to collapse and fracture.

3. Prevention of osteoporosis requires a lifetime of adequate dietary and/or supplemental calcium, weight-bearing exercise to stimulate the bone to deposit calcium, and enough dietary or supplemental vitamin D.

4. At menopause, the keys to preventing osteoporosis are estrogen replacement therapy and continuation of ample calcium intake.

5. Several disorders and medications such as thyroid hormone, tobacco, and steroids accelerate the development of osteoporosis.

6. Every menopausal woman should have routine densitometry done to assess the calcium content of her bones.

7. There are several new drugs you can take to slow the thinning of the bones and even reverse osteoporosis. The most important new agents now available are alendronate (Fosamax), calcitonin (Miacalcin), preferably in the nasal-spray form, and etidronate (Didronel).

8. Raloxifene has both pro- and anti-estrogen effects. It is expected to be as effective against osteoporosis as estrogen, without any of the hormone's adverse effects.

13

PROSTATE ENLARGEMENT

To Pee or Not to Pee—
That Is the Question

At a recent dinner of the New York Heart Association, Diane Sawyer, the noted television anchor, introduced me for an award I was about to receive. She said some very nice things about me and the books I have written. She singled out *Symptoms,* a copy of which she said she keeps by her bed. "Whenever I have something wrong with me, I look it up in *Symptoms* and always find the answer. Why, only this morning I referred to it and discovered that my problem was due to an enlarged prostate."

Either she or my book was wrong! Women have ovaries; men have a prostate. These sex glands respond to the aging process in different ways. At menopause, the ovaries dramatically reduce the amount of hormone (estrogen) and as a result don't make enough for the menstrual cycles to continue, or to prevent osteoporosis, or to maintain a moist vagina. On the other hand, the prostate never makes any hormones, but it enlarges as it ages. There is no way you can prevent either menopause or an enlarged prostate. Every woman will become menopausal as she approaches fifty (no ifs, ands, or buts); 10 percent of men at age thirty, 50 percent over the age of fifty, 80 percent at age seventy, and 90 percent by the time they're eighty-five have an enlarged prostate, a condition called benign prostatic hyperplasia (BPH). (Hyperplasia is the term for increased numbers of normal cells.)

Whether or not your prostate enlarges has nothing to do with how sexually active you are, whether you've had a vasectomy, drink too much, smoke, or are overweight. While these are important risk factors for other disorders, they do not contribute to the enlargement of the prostate. Although the prostate gland does not make any hormones, it does produce the watery fluid in the ejaculate in which the sperm travel and which enhances their motility. This function is under the control of the male hormone, testosterone, which also determines the size of the prostate.

Although BPH has no hormonal consequences, it does affect a man's quality of life. Whereas a woman can ease her menopausal symptoms with hormone replacement, the only thing a man suffering from the symptoms of BPH could do until fairly recently was to have this gland surgically removed. That option is being exercised less and less because there are now several effective medications and procedures that provide relief.

Why an Enlarged Prostate Causes Symptoms

In order to understand the symptoms of BPH and the various treatment options available, you should know something about the structure and location of the prostate gland, and what happens when it enlarges.

The normal prostate gland is the size and shape of a walnut (in its shell) and, like so many other organs, it's wrapped in a capsule. It weighs about twenty grams, and is located in the pelvis just below the urinary bladder. It wraps around the first inch or so of the urethra, the tube that carries urine from the bladder through the penis to its tip. Although we don't know why the prostate enlarges with age, it almost certainly has something to do with testosterone production or activity.

When the prostate gets big enough (it can become the size of a grapefruit), it blocks the flow of urine from the bladder by pressing on the urinary duct passing through it. Since urine can no longer flow freely out of the body, it backs up and distends the urinary bladder. There is also another mechanism contributing to the development of BPH. The prostate gland contains muscle fibers that normally contract and relax. When the prostate enlarges, these muscles squeeze the neck of the urinary bladder, further impeding the outflow of urine. (This is important for you to know because, as you will see, one of the drugs to treat BPH relaxes this muscular constriction and improves urinary flow.)

Symptoms of an Enlarged Prostate

• **A sudden, uncontrollable need to urinate** because the bladder is full and can't handle another drop being made by the kidneys.

• **A weak, interrupted stream** (forget about peeing over a fence like you could when you were young) because the urethra, which determines the size of the stream, is narrowed.

• **Difficulty starting to urinate** (if you're in a hurry or need to pass urine urgently, never stand in line behind an older man in the men's room) because when the bladder gives you the signal to "go," it takes a while for the urine to make it through the constricted urethra.

• **A feeling that you haven't emptied your bladder** after you've ostensibly "finished."

• **Awakening frequently during the night,** as often as every hour or more. Since the kidneys keep sending urine into the bladder, which is already full and can't accommodate any more, you're always getting the signal to "go." Each time you do, you void only the overflow from the bladder, rather than emptying it like someone with a normal-sized prostate does. (The way you void when you take a diuretic is different from that of BPH. The water pill makes you go more often because the kidney is producing more urine, sending it down to the bladder, which fills sooner. Under these circumstances, you pee a large amount, a bladderful, rather than the driblets from overflow in BPH.)

• **Blood in the urine** because the enlarged prostate is also congested. The dilated blood vessels can leak blood into the urine.

• **Burning or painful urination** because the urine can become infected when it sits around in the distended bladder waiting to be eliminated. This gives bacteria a chance to settle down in it and multiply. Urine that's passed after being freshly made and delivered to the bladder for excretion is much less likely to harbor bacteria.

See your doctor if you develop any of the above symptoms since they can be due to causes other than an enlarged prostate. Urinary-tract infection produces many similar symptoms, such as frequency, urgency, and discomfort when voiding even when the prostate is not enlarged; blood in the urine may be due to problems in the kidney or the bladder.

Diagnosing BPH

If you're a middle-aged man or older and suffer from the symptoms listed above, here is what your doctor will do:

• Examine your urine for evidence of infection.
• Perform a digital rectal examination (DRE) to determine the size of the prostate and what it feels like. A cancerous prostate is hard and irregular, in contrast to a benignly enlarged prostate, which is smooth and much softer.

- Obtain a PSA blood test to also help exclude the possibility of cancer. But don't panic if yours comes back somewhat elevated; BPH can also raise the PSA (though not to the same extent as cancer does). Most urologists recommend an ultrasound study and a biopsy of the prostate to evaluate an elevated PSA.
- The next step is to determine what effect the prostatic enlargement is having on your urinary flow. In order to find out, a urine flow-rate test is done. This is a noninvasive measurement of the force, speed, and volume of the urine when you pass it.
- An additional ultrasound examination, in which the scanner is placed on your abdomen, can also be done to see how much urine is actually left in the bladder after you think you've emptied it (this is called the postvoid residual urine test).
- Have your serum creatinine level measured. This is a simple blood test that indicates how well the kidneys are excreting the waste products of metabolism. If you have BPH and urine has been backing up in the bladder, this engorgement may affect the kidneys, distend them, and impair their function.
- If there is still any doubt about the diagnosis or if some other cause is suspected of blocking the urinary flow, a cystoscopy will be done. This is an invasive procedure in which the lower urinary tract can be viewed with a telescope to rule out the presence of a stone, polyp, or tumor.

Treating BPH

Let's assume that you have BPH and the symptoms are bothering you. Don't do anything drastic unless it's interfering with the quality of your life. I have many patients whose only complaint is that they get up two or three times a night. They have no trouble falling back to sleep, and they haven't had any urinary bleeding or infections. I advise them to live with it. But if your symptoms are more severe, there are some treatments that will help.

Until a few years ago, when the diagnosis of BPH was made and your symptoms were disabling, you would almost certainly end up having an operation. The most common surgery involved "reaming out" the prostate with an instrument introduced through the penis into the urethra. The excess tissue surrounding and obstructing this tube was scraped away, increasing the amount of urine that you would be able to pass through it. However, if you were unlucky and your prostate was too big for this procedure, you needed the suprapubic operation. This is full-fledged surgery in which an incision is made in the abdomen and the surgeon goes directly into the pelvis, exposes the prostate, and, under direct vision, removes the obstructing tissue.

Here's how you're apt to be treated these days. First, you'll be given some common-sense advice. If you're up all night peeing, you don't want to aggravate matters by drinking liquids at or near bedtime. That simply adds to the fluid load your kidneys must excrete. Also, if you have to get up frequently at night, put a little night-light in your bathroom rather than turning on the overhead light. It has been suggested that exposure to bright light during the night, even for just a few minutes, stops your brain from making melatonin, the sleep hormone, and may thus make it more difficult for you to return to sleep. If your prostate is inflamed (prostatitis) so that you're not only voiding frequently but it burns when you do, avoid alcohol. Caffeine is a diuretic, so cut down your intake of coffee, tea, soft drinks, and chocolate. Spicy foods make matters worse in some patients, and constipation doesn't help, either. Take a hot bath at bedtime to relax the smooth muscle of the prostate, and try not to sit anywhere for too long, especially on a bicycle seat. Finally, here's a piece of advice you won't find too hard to take: Regular ejaculations ease congestion of the prostate.

Keep in mind that men with a big prostate are at risk for developing acute urinary retention—when you suddenly can't pee at all. The kidney continues to send urine to the bladder, but that's as far as it goes because the large prostate prevents the urine from leaving. The urine load distends the bladder, and you become progressively more uncomfortable. This is a real emergency that requires you go to the nearest emergency room. There, a catheter is introduced into your bladder through the penis and the urine withdrawn. Pseudoephedrine, a decongestant present in many cold remedies, increases the risk of acute urinary retention by causing the smooth muscle in the already enlarged prostate to contract. Antihistamines, so widely used in the treatment of allergic reactions and found in many cough and cold preparations (for no good reason, as far as I'm concerned), weaken the bladder contractions, so that urine tends to be retained. Some medications for the treatment of glaucoma may have a similar effect, so always tell your eye doctor about your prostate problem.

If you have prostate symptoms and your doctor tells you your prostate is at least 40 grams or larger, take *finasteride (Proscar)*. Frankly, it took a long time before I was convinced that this drug works. It does, but you've got to be patient—you won't see its effects overnight.

In 1998, after a four-year trial in over 3,000 men, a single 5-milligram tablet of Proscar taken every day reduced by 57 percent the risk of developing acute urinary retention; it decreased by 55 percent the need for surgery—and it accomplished both these salutary effects without too many side effects. One man in twelve blamed his impotence on Proscar, 6 percent claimed their libido had diminished, and 3 percent said they had a smaller volume of ejaculate. This was a double-blind trial, and it's interesting that after the first year these complaints of impaired sexual function were the same for the placebo group as for those receiving Proscar. The researchers found that the benefits of Proscar became apparent after only four months of treatment. As a result of this landmark study, the FDA has cleared Proscar as the first and only medication to reduce the incidence of acute urinary retention and the need for surgery. There is currently ongoing research to see whether Proscar will also lower the incidence of prostate cancer.

One of the mechanisms that enlarge the prostate is the action of testosterone. (Men who are castrated, for whatever reason, before age forty and so stop producing testosterone, do not develop either cancer or benign enlargement of the prostate.) The active form of this hormone, dihydrotestosterone (DHT), accelerates the growth of normal prostate tissue. Proscar blocks overproduction of DHT and not only prevents further enlargement of the prostate but also causes it to shrink. (The decrease of DHT not only benefits men with prostate enlargement, it can also improve baldness. So in a double whammy, the FDA also approved a weaker strength of Proscar, 1 milligram daily, for the treatment of baldness. The drug is marketed as Propecia.)

Researchers in Europe and practitioners of alternative medicine in this country insist that an *extract of the saw palmetto berry* is cheaper than and as effective as Proscar in controlling the symptoms of prostatism, and that it does so by the same mechanism. They cite several reports in the European literature documenting this effect. However, although saw palmetto relieves symptoms it does not shrink the prostate, which Proscar does do. When saw palmetto alone is not enough, some naturopaths add the herbs pygeum and *Urtica dioica.*

The only advantages of these herbal remedies over Proscar are cost and the fact that they do not lower the level of the PSA, which, you will remember, is what doctors measure in the blood to detect prostate cancer. Proscar reduces the PSA level by about half and thus renders this test less useful as an indicator of prostate cancer.

If you're getting up every hour or so to void, you don't have to wait for months for the Proscar or saw palmetto to work. Medications called *alpha-adrenergic blockers* *(Hytrin, Cardura, Flomax)* can provide relief quickly. They work on the muscular component of BPH described earlier. When the prostate muscle clamps down on the outlet of the urinary bladder, it prevents the outflow of urine from that organ. The alpha-adrenergic blockers release this spasm. Taking them at bedtime really does reduce the number of times you'll need to get up at night. However, a word of caution is in order: All the adrenergic blockers except Flomax lower blood pressure and are especially prone to causing postural hypotension. That means that when you change position from lying to sitting, or sitting to standing, your blood pressure can drop precipitously. So the very first night you start one of these pills, take the smallest dose and change position very slowly and gradually. Of course, if you have BPH and high blood pressure, these agents kill two birds with one stone and may allow you to lower the dose of your other blood-pressure medications. Nasal stuffiness is another side effect of these adrenergic blockers.

Suppose that Proscar and Hytrin have eased your symptoms, but you're still worn out during the day because of the sleep you've lost during the night going to the john. Your doctor raises the possibility of surgery. He or she will tell you that 400,000 transurethral resections (TURPs—that's the one through the penis) are done in this country every year, and that this operation remains the gold standard for the relief of prostatic obstruction. That's true, but in the past six or seven years several other options have become available. At the moment, most of them are being done only in large medical centers. Ask your doctor about them. They may be worth a trip. These less invasive techniques don't require hospitalization and can be done with only local anesthesia. Results are pretty good, although probably not as long lasting as the more invasive TURP. In my opinion, however, the benefit of an easier, quicker, less risky procedure outweighs the drawback of earlier recurrence. Here are some of the more widely used of these minimally invasive techniques:

Microwave therapy (transurethral microwave thermotherapy or TUMT) is the most promising and popular of these techniques. In this procedure, a catheter is inserted into the urethra through the penis and directs microwaves into the prostate, heating and killing the excess tissue. The treatment takes about an hour. The FDA approved this device, called the Prostatron, in 1997.

Another form of local therapy is called *transurethral needle ablation (TUNA)*, in which a scope is inserted into the urethra and two small needles are introduced into the surrounding prostate tissue. The gland is then zapped with radiofrequency energy. The FDA has also approved TUNA.

Both TUMT and TUNA are outpatient procedures, and although you may need a catheter left in place for a few days, you can go home and back to work the next day (unless, of course, you're a bathing suit model). The TURP procedure, on the other hand, usually involves a hospital stay of about three days. Improvement after a TUMT or TUNA is not quite as dramatic as it is after a TURP, and the long-term effectiveness of either of these techniques is uncertain, but both do offer relief for at least two years.

Laser prostatectomy is also an outpatient procedure, but it requires general anesthesia, and you'll be wearing a catheter for the next week to ten days. A tiny laser is inserted into the penis and directs its beam into the prostate tissue, causing only minimal bleeding. Most urologists with whom I have spoken don't give this laser approach the same high marks as the TUMT.

A newer procedure known as *transurethral electrovaporization of the prostate (TEVP)* vaporizes excess prostate tissue with an electric current. TEVP requires general or spinal anesthesia and hospitalization for a few days. As is the case with TUNA, you may experience permanent "dry" ejaculation after TEVP—the semen is discharged back into the bladder and does not come out of the penis. There is a growing belief that TEVP will eventually replace TURP because it results in fewer complications, less bleeding, lower cost, and fewer days in the hospital.

A *transurethral incision of the prostate (TUIP)* can be done if the enlargement of the gland is not too great. In this operation, pressure on the urethra is relieved by several small cuts in the tissue compressing it.

A few years ago, *ballooning of the prostate* was the rage. It's very much like an angioplasty of the coronary arteries in the heart. The balloon is inserted into the urethra, where it is inflated to dilate the constricted portion. Long-term results have not been good and the procedure is no longer widely used.

The latest technique, and one that is still very experimental, is the application of *high-intensity ultrasound* to destroy prostate tissue. It's similar to microwave therapy and is done in much the same way.

The urological community is not in agreement as to which of these procedures is the best. At the moment, however, many prefer the TEVP to the TURP. Although the latter gives the most predictable long-term results, it does involve an operation, which may present some risk, especially to older men who are in poor health.

What to Remember about Prostate Enlargement

1. Enlargement of the prostate (BPH) may begin as early as the thirties, and affects most men by the time they're seventy.
2. Symptoms of BPH are due to: (a) obstruction of urinary outflow caused by narrowing of the urethra by the enlarged prostate gland; and (b) spasm of smooth muscle in the gland.
3. BPH does not lead to prostate cancer or affect sexual function.
4. Fewer cases of BPH now require surgery because of the availability of newer drugs such as Proscar and beta-adrenergic blockers such as Hytrin, Cardura, and Flomax.
5. When drugs do not relieve symptoms, several new, less invasive techniques are available to remove excessive prostate tissue.

14

AGING SKIN

A Dry and Flaky Chapter

Beauty is only skin deep, but the appearance of your skin is the standard by which people judge health and biological age. No one sees your liver, lungs, kidneys, or heart, but your face is always on display. Even if you're full of vim, vigor, and vitality and never felt better in your life, the rest of the world considers you old if your face is lined, wrinkled, the skin is loose around the neck, baggy under the eyes, and full of crow's-feet and brown spots. That inspired the story of the elderly man who died while vacationing in Florida. After his remains were returned to New York, one of his friends viewing the tanned corpse in the casket declared, "Look at that tan! That's living!"

The skin is the largest organ of the body—and it's an important one. Even though we tend to think of it as only a cover for the more important stuff inside, its structure is complex, and it does much more than prevent what's inside the body from spilling out. Skin senses and regulates body temperature; it retains heat when it's cold outside and eliminates it when the weather is hot; it alerts us to pain or pressure and is the mirror of many internal diseases, allergies, and other adverse reactions.

In this chapter we will explore how and why skin ages, and how to slow down the process.

Changes in the appearance and character of your skin are inevitable as you grow older, but their severity depends on your genes, your lifestyle, and your habits. The most superficial portion of the skin is the epidermis, whose upper layer is called the stratum corneum. You can forget that name, but remember that its functions are to retain the moisture in skin and to prevent toxic substances from getting into the body.

When Skin Ages

- The dermis, or internal layer of the skin just below the epidermis, contains glands, follicles, nerves, blood vessels, and elastin (the fibers in the dermis that make the skin resilient). As skin ages it loses some of its elastin. You know how when you pinch a baby's bottom the skin promptly snaps back into place. However, when you pinch the skin of someone over sixty (not necessarily his or her bottom), it stretches and falls back much more slowly.

- Collagen, the protein that supports and gives skin its body, also decreases with age. As a result, your skin is eventually about 20 percent less thick than when you were younger.

- The blood supply to the skin decreases with age too;

there are fewer blood vessels and their walls are thinner and more fragile. This leaves the skin less well
nourished and more vulnerable to injury, infection,
and bruising.

- In young people injured skin is promptly replaced by
  new tissue. A sunburn is the best example of this re-
  newal process. After the scorched, dead skin peels,
  new, healthy skin forms. However, in older people, the
  ability of the skin cells to reproduce is compromised,
  and they have a shorter life span. So as you get older,
  it takes longer for your skin to heal than when you
  were young.

- Sweat glands in the skin decrease in number with age,
  and its sebaceous glands make less oil, so that the skin
  is not as moist or as well lubricated. It then becomes
  dry and itchy, especially in winter.

What Aging Skin Looks Like

- **Aging skin is thin, dry, wrinkled, discolored,
  fragile, inelastic,** and, in some very old people, almost
  transparent, like parchment.

- **Tags** may form in areas where the skin is very loose
  and/or subjected to friction (the groin, the armpits, and
  under the breasts in females). These tags, little pieces of
  skin that you're tempted to pull off, usually appear in
  women in their forties and in men some ten years later.
  They are rarely malignant, but check them out anyway
  because skin cancers sometimes masquerade as skin tags.

• **Seborrheic keratoses** are brown raised spots that look like warts. Though not a threat to your health, they can be cosmetically embarrassing. Your dermatologist can scrape them off, or remove them with liquid nitrogen.

• **Actinic keratoses** are premalignant and should be removed, usually by freezing with liquid nitrogen. Don't mistake them for seborrheic keratoses. Actinic keratoses are skin lesions in areas that have been chronically exposed to the sun—they are most often seen in blondes and redheads. They resemble little warts but are rough and sometimes hard to the touch; they tend to be dark gray, unlike seborrheic keratoses, which are generally brown.

• **"Age" or liver spots** (doctors call them lentigines) are large, flat, irregular, discolored areas most commonly seen on portions of the skin that are exposed to the sun most often: the face, the back of the hands, and the feet.

I have no idea why they're called liver spots since they have nothing to do with the liver. And don't waste your money on any "fading" creams that promise to remove them; they don't work. I have seen several malignant melanomas mistaken for these harmless liver spots, so always have a dermatologist take a look at them if there's ever any question.

• **Little bright red areas called** *cherry angiomas* begin to appear on your skin when you become middle-aged, and are ultimately present in about 85 percent of healthy older people. They are more common on the torso rather than the limbs, and are nothing more than tiny dilated blood vessels, a harmless manifestation of age.

• **Have you noted areas of bruising, or black or blue marks,** especially on your arms and legs? These are called purpura, and they develop in older people whose skin is thin, inelastic, and has lost its fat and connective tissues. As a result, underlying blood vessels are not well supported and are thus vulnerable to injury. Purpura is worsened by exposure to sun. However, let your doctor know if any of these marks appear in areas of the skin that are covered, or if they are accompanied by bleeding elsewhere in the body.

All these "natural" consequences of aging skin—the loss of elastin and collagen, the slowed reproduction of skin cells, the reduction in the number of sweat glands, and the decreased secretion of oil (sebum) from the sebaceous glands—are accelerated and aggravated by exposure to sun, emotional stress, poor nutrition, recurrent fluctuations in weight, alcohol abuse, pollution, and cigarette smoking. The most important of these risk factors are the sun's rays.

The Hazards of Sun

Before I pan the tan, let me point out that sun is not all bad. Its rays can be therapeutic for anyone with psoriasis, arthritis, and some cases of asthma. Also, the skin needs a certain amount of sunlight in order to produce the vitamin D that protects our bones (but you're better off getting this vitamin from your pharmacy than from the sun).

The bad news is that solar hazards far outweigh the benefits. Many nondermatological conditions such as cold sores, chicken pox, and lupus are aggravated by sunlight. Basking and broiling in the sun is the single most important cause of the wrinkling, yellowing, drying, coarsening, and blotching that characterize aging skin, not to mention skin cancer. Dry skin also predisposes you to other dermatological disorders such as eczema, and thin skin leads to pressure sores in the elderly.

It's ironic that while we spend millions of dollars on creams, face-lifts, collagen injections, and other cosmetic procedures to smooth our wrinkles, cover our brown spots, moisturize our dermis, and tighten the various sagging and drooping areas of our bodies, at least one-third of us continue to seek out the sun to get a "good tan" (an oxymoron if I ever heard one). We do so because sitting in the sun feels so good, and, in our culture, a bronzed body symbolizes fitness, health, and the good life. Let me confess: I myself happen to be one of those short-sighted sun worshipers. Since I spend most of my time indoors, I chronically have a ghastly pallor, and my patients are constantly telling me how pale I look. They probably wonder whether I'm anemic and/or suffering from some underlying illness. Happily, I've solved my problem. I'll let you in on my secret, but ask that you please keep it confidential: I avoid the sun, but every third or fourth night I apply a bronzer on my face—just enough to remove the pasty look. The downside is that an obvious "tan" prompts people to ask me where I've been. It's hard to answer that question during the winter in New York when I haven't missed a day's work.

If you're an active sun worshiper or have an outdoor job, your skin will ultimately become tough and leathery, making you look fifteen to twenty years older than you are. As little as five to fifteen minutes of strong sunlight every second day is enough to cause obvious photoaging of your skin (even on foggy or cloudy days, because up to 80 percent of untraviolet rays can get through the clouds). If you come to your senses in time and stop sunbathing, the skin can regain some of the lost collagen.

The sun is hazardous to everyone, but especially if you're Caucasian, if your skin is fair and burns easily, and your hair is light in color. Orientals are somewhat less vulnerable, and African Americans tolerate the sun best. In addition to the light that you see and feel, the sun emits invisible ultraviolet (UV) rays that weaken the elastin in the dermis. They also lead to the release of enzymes that dissolve the collagen that supports the skin and keeps it taut. There's yet another harmful solar effect. Skin contains melanocytes, cells that allow us to tan, not so that we look beautiful, but to protect the skin from injury by the ultraviolet light. We lose about 20 percent of these pigment-producing cells every ten years after the age of thirty. As this total decreases, so does the ability to ward off the sun's harmful rays. Older people don't tan as evenly because they have fewer melanocytes. Those that remain tend to clump together and make the final tan, such as it is, irregular.

The best way to prevent sun damage to the skin is to avoid excessive exposure beginning early in life. Don't visit tanning parlors during the winter months to maintain your color. Ultraviolet rays from a machine may be more harmful than those from the sun. Here are some guidelines to follow whenever you go outdoors in sunny weather for any length of time:

- Avoid the sun when its rays are strongest, between ten in the morning and three in the afternoon.
- If you live in a sunny clime and spend time outdoors playing tennis, gardening, hiking, or whatever else you enjoy doing, use protective clothing that's loose, light-colored, and tightly woven. Wet clothes that cling to your skin permit penetration by UV rays.
- Beach umbrellas don't protect against UV light that bounces off the water and sand.
- If you're a skier, remember that snow reflects 80 percent of the sun's rays. (I got one of my deepest tans on the slopes of Saint-Moritz in Switzerland one winter.) It's easier to get burned at high altitudes because the thin atmosphere does not block out UV rays as effectively.
- Wear a hat with a large brim and a flap that covers the neck, too.
- A long-sleeved shirt will filter out about 50 percent of the ultraviolet rays, and an undershirt further increases that protection to 70 percent.
- Sunglasses with UV filters are also important (see Chapter 19).

- Apply sunscreen liberally to exposed areas of the body about a half hour before you go outside (even if it's cloudy or you plan to be in the shade), and reapply it after swimming or perspiring heavily. An SPF (sun protection factor) of 15 drops to only 7 if you don't put on enough of it. The higher the SPF the better, but don't settle for anything less than 15. The basic ingredient in most sunscreens that keeps the harmful short ultraviolet rays (UV-B) from your skin is PABA (para-amino-benzoic acid). We used to think that only the UV-B mattered, but we now know that UV-A, the longer rays, are also harmful. Newer broad-spectrum sunscreens contain oxybenzone and Parsol 1789 (look for this information on the label) that block those longer UV-A wavelengths too. One final note: A sun reflector can result in serious burns to the delicate tissues of the eyelids, ears, and face. Never, ever use one.

Treating Skin That's Aged

The quest for a youthful skin is a multibillion-dollar industry in the United States. The approaches range from topical creams, oils, and lotions to a variety of cosmetic surgical procedures. Here are some useful tips on skin care.

Don't shower or bathe more than once a day if your skin is dry; the hotter the water, the more drying it is. Use very mild soap such as Dove or Basis that won't dry or irritate your skin. I also recommend one that's "superfatted," nonsudsing, and cleans the skin without removing its natural oils. Don't douse with astringent perfumes or use excessive amounts of antiperspirants. Be careful with bath oils: They make the skin feel moist, at least temporarily, but they also leave the bathtub slippery, so you can fall getting into or out of it.

Dab your skin after a bath or a shower—don't rub it—and leave it a little damp. Then apply some lanolin, mineral oil, or jojoba oil to help retain the moisture. If your skin is cracked and inflamed, use a mild topical cortisone preparation. Winter is the worst time for dry skin because the dry air and heated rooms reduce the humidity of the skin. Keep your home, especially your bedroom, as humid as possible, with a humidifier if necessary. Your hands need special protection; they are exposed not only to the elements (the most important of which is sun) but to other physical irritants as well. So wear gloves when washing the dishes, gardening, or working at anything that exposes them to chemicals or irritants.

Dry skin is vulnerable to irritation and itching. Coffee, alcohol, spicy foods, and, believe it or not, too much exercise can all make matters worse. Before attributing your itchiness to aging skin, remember that many diseases such as diabetes, hypothyroidism, and disorders of the liver, kidney, or gallbladder can also cause itching. So can a variety of drugs, especially diuretics (water pills). If your skin is dry for any reason, wear cotton next to it rather than wool or some other rough fabric.

COSMETIC MOISTURIZERS

Cosmetic moisturizers are the most heavily advertised treatments for dry and itching skin. However, virtually every one of them moistens the skin only temporarily. None cure; they conceal but don't heal. These products sell more hype and hope than help. There is not much to choose among them, except for scent and "feel," regardless of the price. The least costly, unscented, and unmedicated products such as simple petrolatum (Vaseline) are as effective as any. Even so, don't use any of them too much. Mineral oil can cause the skin to break out and in large amounts can dissolve the skin's own natural oils, leaving it even drier than before.

Several of my patients enjoy a drying *facial mask* every week or two. They find it pleasant and relaxing, and it leaves their skin looking and feeling good for a few hours. The mask makes the skin tingle and tight, and creates the illusion of a therapeutic effect. There is none. A few hours after the mask is removed, you're back to square one. *Albumin,* the main ingredient in most of these facial masks, is touted as a wrinkle remover. Although it does create a film that hides the wrinkles temporarily, it doesn't remove them. *Bentonite,* a naturally occurring mineral, is another substance commonly present in facial-mask formulas. When mixed with liquid, it forms an impermeable gel that some dermatologists worry may keep oxygen away from the skin. *Kaolin,* a clay that originally came from Mount Gaoling in China, is another ingredient sometimes added to facial masks to create the feeling of tightness. Its drying and dehydrating properties keep needed oxygen from the skin—not a good thing. If these facial masks make you happy, it's okay to have them from time to time. They're a lot safer than some other therapies and a whole lot better than a suntan. But don't expect any lasting change in the appearance of your skin.

Here's the scientific scoop on some of the other ingredients in various "miracle" cosmetics. Look carefully at the labels for the following:

Biotin: You'll read that this vitamin is absolutely necessary for healthy skin and hair. While it's true that biotin deficiency in rats and other experimental animals makes their scalps greasy and may even leave them bald, humans are not fur-bearing animals, and biotin deficiency is extremely rare. The bottom line? You're wasting your money when you pay for biotin in a cosmetic.

Elastin is present in some skin-care products, the assumption being that since it's lost from the skin as we get older, we should put some back in a cream or lotion. Unfortunately, the elastin you apply to your skin doesn't penetrate it. Even though it does help retain some moisture, I wouldn't pay extra for it.

A *humectant* is something that draws moisture. *Glycerin,* one of the many humectants, is a combination of water and fat that's added to many creams and lotions to help them spread easily and prevent them from evaporating and drying out. The problem with glycerin is that unless the humidity is over 65 percent, it sucks the moisture *from* the skin, drying it from the inside out. So use glycerin only when it's sticky outdoors and raining!

Many of my patients and friends who have skin allergies will not buy any cosmetic that isn't *hypoallergenic*. This term is a triumph of obfuscation and modern advertising. "Hypo" means "less." Something that's hypoallergenic is supposed to contain fewer allergens—things that can provoke an allergic reaction. But the term *hypoallergenic* has never been defined, no one really knows what it means, and there are no federal guidelines or definitions. So we're left with "hypo" or "less," without knowing "less" than what, and by how much.

Placental extracts are another example of advertising hype. After all, the pitch goes, what can be better for old adults than a placenta that nourishes the embryo? It should do wonders for the skin, shouldn't it? The truth is it does nothing at all.

Royal bee jelly is another advertising triumph. Great for the queen bee, worthless for humans. And if it's left lying around for longer than two weeks, it won't help even the queen bee!

THERAPEUTIC MOISTURIZERS

Therapeutic moisturizers are generally more effective than the simple cosmetic moisturizers. The most extensively researched among them contain tretinoin, alpha-hydroxy acids (AHA—products with alcohol and a variety of acids), and beta-hydroxy acids (BHA-containing salicylic acids).

Tretinoin (marketed as Retin-A, Renova), belongs to a class of compounds derived from vitamin A. It's very effective against acne. It has also become popular for treating aging skin. Some dermatologists believe that these retinoids may also help prevent skin cancer. Tretinoin does result in some cosmetic improvement: It gives better facial color, somewhat softer skin texture, and renders fine wrinkles less apparent. (It doesn't do much for deeper expression lines or wrinkles.) Tretinoin probably works by neutralizing collagen-destroying enzymes that are produced in the dermis by the sun's rays. It also increases the number of capillaries (small blood vessels) in the skin that bring more oxygen and other nutrients to the area. Although Tretinoin improves sundamaged skin, I'm not convinced that it restores loss of elasticity.

The downside to using Retin-A is that it can also make the skin peel and turn red, scaly, puffy, and blistered. This is especially apt to happen after you've been in the sun. So when you're using Retin-A, keep out of the sun and avoid any topical products that contain sulfur, resorcinol, salicylic acid, or benzoyl peroxide.

Tretinoin comes in several different strengths, depending on your skin type and the severity of your problem. It's applied once a day, and takes at least twelve weeks to work. Don't be surprised if your wrinkles return after you stop using it. You can safely use Retin-A for up to twenty years.

Alpha-hydroxy acids (AHA) slow the aging skin process, minimize fine wrinkles, cause dead skin to shed, open the pores (that's why they help acne, too), and even lighten some aging spots. The natural sources of AHA are fruit, sugarcane, and dairy products; commercial preparations are available as lotions, solutions, and creams. The most effective ones contain lactic or glycolic acids. These preparations vary in strength—the weakest contain less than 12 percent, even as little as 1 percent, and can be bought over-the-counter; the strongest contain 70 percent and require a doctor's prescription. We used to think that only the prescription strengths work, but recent research has shown that the weaker products are also effective. (If you're using either Retin-A or AHA, make sure to apply a sunblock or sunscreen with an SPF of at least 17 before you go outdoors, to protect against increased vulnerability to the sun caused by both these products.)

Beta-hydroxy acids (BHA) have essentially the same mechanism as the alpha variety: They accelerate the cell turnover of the skin surface. Many dermatologists believe that the beta-hydroxy acids actually get into the pores and also exfoliate the skin—that is, remove the dead superficial layer—a little more deeply than do the alpha-hydroxy acids. They're also less irritating, and because they contain salicylic acid (a derivative of aspirin), they also have an anti-inflammatory effect on the skin. If you've got some little whiteheads superimposed on your aging skin, the beta-hydroxy formulation will help you more. Some enthusiasts report that the combination of AHA and BHA yields better results than either alone.

SKIN PROCEDURES THAT HELP

Given the limitations of cosmetics, you may want to consider some of the procedures that can remove the stigma of age. These include:

A *skin peel*, or resurfacing, is a modification of dermabrasion and usually requires pretreatment with Retin-A or AHA. Chemicals such as phenol or trichloracetic acid (TCA) or a carbon dioxide (CO_2) laser beam strip away dead and aging skin. This presumably encourages the body to form new layers and to make more collagen to fill out some of the wrinkles. Phenol and TCA sometimes cause excessive pigmentation of the skin, so that you may have to add a bleaching agent, such as hydroquinone. Such hyperpigmentation is not only unsightly, it can be dangerous too.

Laser beams can burn away the damaged superficial layers of skin, leaving a new, pink surface. This procedure usually causes a burning sensation for a while, and the newly formed skin remains red and watery for days.

Chemical and laser peeling of the skin can produce impressive long-term improvement in finer lines and wrinkles. However, if your problem is loose skin, you'll need a face-lift.

There are several different kinds of *face-lifts*—nipping, tucking, collagen injections—all calculated to make you look younger. *Collagen injections* last no more than a year, after which the collagen usually breaks down and the wrinkles return. (Don't confuse the injections with *topical collagen* in creams and lotions. All the advertising hype notwithstanding, the stuff you put on the skin is a protein that doesn't penetrate its surface because the molecule is too large to get into the epidermis. It may, in fact, do more harm by trapping the toxins in the skin and keeping oxygen out.)

A face-lift can do wonders for you but may also leave you taut, scarred, and artificial looking. (A celebrated case in the New York divorce courts at the time of this writing featured a woman ridiculed in the press as the "Bride of Wildenstein," a wealthy socialite who'd had so much plastic surgery her face had lost almost all its elasticity.) Unfortunately, in our relentless search for the fountain of youth, we often attack even minor changes in the skin with such zeal that we lose the charm and character that some "aging" characteristics confer. There are too many among us who look alike, with tight and expressionless faces, the result of cosmetic surgery done in the name of rejuvenation. Even when successful, the benefit of most face-lifts is usually temporary. After a few years, most people revert to the appearance commensurate with their age.

The incision in the classic face-lift is hidden behind the ear or in the scalp. It tightens the loose skin of the face and neck but does not affect the eyes or the forehead.

Blepharoplasty or *eyelid tightening* removes loose skin under the eyes, as well as the excess fat present in the bags or pouches. Deep creases in your forehead may require a *forehead lift*, which removes excess skin and tightens muscles with an incision hidden in the scalp (hidden, of course, only if you have the hair for it).

MISCELLANEOUS SKIN THERAPIES

Topical vitamin C, an antioxidant now available as a skin cream, is absorbed by the skin and is said to facilitate skin repair and to increase the natural formation of collagen. The product with which I am most familiar is marketed as Cell-C, but there are others. It's too early for me to be sure how well this topical vitamin works, but it sounds good theoretically.

If you're menopausal, consider *estrogen replacement therapy* (ERT) for younger-looking skin. Women have known for years that this hormone slows the aging process in the skin (and many other organs too). But there is now measurable, scientific proof that it does so. In a recent study of some 3,800 women done by researchers at the University of California in Los Angeles, those who took estrogen either topically (in a cream or ointment) or by mouth were 25 percent less likely to have dry skin, and had 30 percent fewer wrinkles compared to nonusers. The beneficial effect of this hormone is probably due to the fact that it increases the collagen content of the skin. The all-round benefits of estrogen— its favorable impact on osteoporosis, heart attack, stroke, Alzheimer's, sexuality, and the sense of well-being—are so overwhelming that a younger-looking skin is simply icing on the cake. Unfortunately, a few women who take estrogen develop acne, and in some with a dark complexion, this hormone may cause blotching of the skin.

According to one theory, skin ages because of a deficiency of oxygen. As circulation is decreased, the skin receives fewer vital nutrients. That's presumably why cigarettes, which constrict the blood vessels, accelerate the aging of skin. If this theory is correct, then, theoretically, a hyperbaric oxygen chamber, which delivers oxygen under high pressure, should solve the problem. But such machines are not universally available (there are only some 400 through the United States), they're expensive, and they're impractical for this purpose. Some doctors think the next best thing is *topical hydrogen peroxide emulsion,* which supposedly delivers as much as four atmospheres of hyperbaric oxygen. Adding vitamins C and E to the hydrogen peroxide is said to make it even more effective. I have seen very little documentation of the benefits of hydrogen peroxide, and I would strongly suggest that you check with your dermatologist before you apply it.

The other day when I walked in to my examining room, I found my patient, a forty-five-year old woman, sitting there making the strangest faces. To my relief, she wasn't demented or disturbed; she was merely practicing *facial exercises* to get rid of her wrinkles. She was very disappointed when I told her this was the wrong thing to do. Making such facial movements in public not only raises questions about your sanity, they also actually produce the very wrinkles they're supposed to remove.

What to Remember about Aging Skin

1. The skin is the largest organ in the body and is as vulnerable to the aging process as any other organ.

2. As we age, our skin becomes thinner, loses its supporting tissues, and dries out due to decreased blood supply and decreased production of oily substances.

3. The natural aging process of the skin is greatly accelerated by several factors, the most important of which are sun, stress, genetic factors, and smoking.

4. There are several important steps you can take to slow down the thinning and drying of the skin, and to protect it against the sun. These include applying sunscreen, wearing protective clothing, and, most important of all, avoiding exposure when the sun's rays are strongest.

5. Virtually all cosmetic moisturizers provide only temporary relief from dry skin and itching and do not address the underlying causes.

6. Therapeutic moisturizers can reduce fine wrinkles, but not the deeper furrows.

7. Skin-peeling procedures, both chemical and using laser beams, can improve the appearance of the aging skin.

8. Various cosmetic surgical procedures are the only definitive way to restore the youthful look, but these are not always successful.

15

STROKE

Brain Attack!

Stroke is the third leading cause of death in this country. It affects more than 500,000 people every year, of whom 150,000 die. There are 3 million stroke survivors among us, 2 million of whom are permanently paralyzed, are speech-impaired, or are disabled by a variety of other neurological problems. There probably isn't a family in the United States that hasn't been touched by stroke. The cost of this illness in human tragedy and shattered lives is incalculable; in terms of money it amounts to $30 billion a year.

The incidence of stroke dropped dramatically between 1970 and 1990, but that trend appears to have ended, and, inexplicably, the number of nonfatal attacks is on the rise. The good news is that the many controllable risk factors that have been identified, along with the many revolutionary advances in treatment, have reduced the permanent disability from a stroke.

There are still many preconceived ideas about stroke that are either outdated or just plain wrong. For example, half of the ninety-eight students at a university in this country, when asked to list all the factors they thought could lead to a stroke, replied that stress was the most important one. Stress doesn't help, but it's by no means an important cause of stroke; only four students knew that diabetics are especially prone to stroke, and only one-third were aware that cigarette smoking is a major cause. You may excuse these youngsters their ignorance because stroke is, after all, largely a disease of older people, and these kids have more pressing problems on their minds. However, that kind of thinking is dangerous because although most strokes do affect the elderly, the stage is set when we're young. It behooves *everyone at every age* to be aware of the important risk factors. If you don't control them in time, you may wind up with a stroke much sooner than you expected.

Kids may not be as well informed about strokes as they should be, but surely most adults are. Surprise! Would you believe that in another recent study, only a small percentage of patients *who'd already had a stroke* were familiar with its symptoms, causes, and prevention? Nearly half of these patients, *while still in the hospital,* did not even realize that something had happened to their brain! Fully 10 percent thought that they'd had some kind of heart attack; another 40 percent had no clue as to what hit them.

Apparently, what little most people do know about stroke comes from their friends and family; only 2 percent learn about it from a medical professional. In this chapter, you will find virtually all the information you need to understand how and why strokes happen, the symptoms, how to control the risk factors, and what treatments offer the best chance of recovery.

What Is a Stroke?

The brain contains billions of brain cells, all of which require constant nutrition. This is provided by blood from a network of arteries that surround and penetrate the brain and that branch into progressively smaller vessels. The tiniest of these, called capillaries, deliver oxygen and other nutrients to the innermost recesses of the brain. When this blood supply is suddenly cut off, cells in the affected area of the brain whose survival depends on it, die within minutes. Such tissue starvation, which resembles what happens to cardiac muscle during a heart attack, is a "brain attack"—and is called a "stroke."

A stroke is usually instantaneous, and its symptoms either clear up completely or become progressively more severe, causing paralysis or death. There's no way, at its onset, to predict what course a stroke will take. So once the telltale symptoms start, you should always assume the worst and get medical help immediately. Making the right diagnosis and initiating treatment right away can mean the difference between complete recovery and permanent paralysis—between life and death. Most people know to get to the nearest emergency room when they suspect a heart attack. *It's just as critical to do so when you think you may be having a brain attack.*

Symptoms of Stroke

The symptoms of a stroke, and their severity, depend on what part of the brain has been deprived of blood, how large an area is involved, and how quickly treatment is started. Suspect a stroke whenever you *suddenly* experience any of the following:

- Weakness or numbness of the face, arm, or leg on one side of the body
- Severe headache with no known or apparent cause
- Loss of speech, or trouble talking or understanding what is being said
- Dimming or loss of vision
- Unexplained dizziness, unsteadiness, or sudden falls, especially associated with any of the other symptoms listed above

The key word here is *sudden*. If symptoms continue for at least fifteen minutes, call your doctor or get to an emergency room—fast. If you wait until the next day because you don't think it's serious, you will lose a treatment opportunity that can save your life. It's better to be safe than sorry.

About a third of all strokes are preceded days, weeks, or months by one or more "ministrokes" or "strokelets." You may feel a sudden weakness of an arm or a leg, or slurring of speech, or a loss of vision that lasts a few minutes or hours and clears up completely within twenty-four hours. Such attacks, called transient ischemic attacks (TIAs)—"ischemia" means decreased blood flow—are the forerunners of a larger stroke. Should you have one of these warnings, call your doctor immediately. Whether it turns out to be a TIA or a full-blown stroke can only be determined by hindsight. Don't be tempted to think these symptoms are "nothing" just because they disappeared completely. They're waiting for the next round—and the knockout blow. Tell your doctor about them without fail.

How Strokes Happen

The blood supply to the brain can be interrupted suddenly in two different ways. The first, and more common, mechanism, is a clot that obstructs the flow of blood within an artery. This clot may either develop in the artery itself (thrombosis) or reach it from some other part of the body. Such a clot is called an embolus. Whatever the mechanism, such blockages, called ischemic strokes, are responsible for 70 to 80 percent of all brain attacks.

The second main category of stroke is "hemorrhagic," and occurs when an artery bursts inside the brain. Here are the various mechanisms that can lead to both the obstructive and the hemorrhagic strokes:

CEREBRAL THROMBOSIS (WHEN THE CLOT FORMS LOCALLY)

A blood clot (thrombosis) that suddenly blocks the flow of blood in a brain artery or in one of the vessels in the neck that carries blood to the brain (carotid artery in the front, vertebral artery in the back) commonly forms at the site of an arteriosclerotic plaque. This "hardening" of the artery has been going on for months or years, and the stroke is the final chapter in a long story of vascular disease. It usually occurs at night or early in the morning, when blood flow through the narrowed artery is at its lowest. The most important risk factors for plaque formation are: high blood pressure, cigarette smoking, poorly controlled diabetes, and excess body weight.

CEREBRAL EMBOLISM

Five to 15 percent of strokes result from an embolism, the obstruction of a cerebral artery by a blood clot (embolus) that *originated elsewhere in the body* and made its way to the brain in the bloodstream. The severity of an embolic stroke depends on the size of the brain artery it has occluded. Remember that embolism is rarely a single event. When you have one, you can assume that more clots are on the way. Incidentally, clots to the brain travel only in arteries, not veins. Those that form in the varicose veins of your legs and break off end up in the lungs and not in the brain.

Emboli to the brain can originate in several different locations. A common and important source is the heart. Within the first few days after a heart attack, a clot can form inside the left ventricle, the main cardiac cavity. When the heart contracts, a small piece of the clot leaves the heart, enters the circulation, and ends up anywhere arteries go—to the eye (causing blindness), to the spleen (giving pain in the abdomen), to the kidneys (producing blood in the urine), or to the brain (resulting in a stroke).

A certain kind of irregular cardiac rhythm, called atrial fibrillation, is a more common source of clots from the heart. Atrial fibrillation is present in about 5 percent of people over the age of sixty-five and accounts for 80,000 of the half-million strokes every year. This rhythm disturbance is more than just a skipped or an extra beat or even a rapid, regular heart rate. A fibrillating heart beat is wildly irregular, and usually (though not always) reflects some kind of underlying heart disease or sometimes an overactive thyroid gland. Occasionally, there is no apparent reason for the fibrillation. Whatever the cause, when the heart fibrillates, tiny clots form within it and these can then travel to parts unknown—including the brain.

Emboli can also originate on the heart valves. The guilty valve may be one of your own that has been diseased by rheumatic fever or an artificial one implanted surgically. These tiny clots adhere to the valve and then break off; they can lodge in the brain and cause a stroke, or travel to other organs such as the kidneys or the legs.

Emboli can also form within a cardiac aneurysm (a ballooning of the heart muscle damaged by a major heart attack) as the blood swirls around within them. A small clot is squeezed out of the heart during one of its contractions, lodges in and obstructs a brain artery—and results in a stroke.

Clots may also break off an arteriosclerotic plaque that has developed within the carotids, the large arteries in the neck leading to the brain. Your doctor can detect the presence of such a plaque when he or she listens to your neck with a stethoscope. Blood flowing through the narrowed artery generates a sound called a "bruit" (the French word for "noise"). If you have a bruit in your carotid, you should have a noninvasive ultrasound (Doppler) test done (see below). In fact, I recommend this procedure to every patient over the age of sixty-five in order to detect silent obstruction of the carotids. This procedure indicates whether a plaque is present and whether it is large enough to require removal.

BLEEDING INTO THE BRAIN (HEMORRHAGIC STROKE)

Ten percent of strokes are hemorrhagic, that is, due to the rupture of an artery in or around the brain that spills blood into the surrounding brain tissue. This is called an intra-cerebral hemorrhage. When a blood vessel on the surface of the brain bleeds into the space between the brain and the skull, it's referred to as a subarachnoid hemorrhage. The most common cause of arterial rupture is a weakening of the vessel wall by the incessant pounding of untreated high blood pressure.

Although hypertension is a common cause of bursting arterial walls, a head injury can do it too. Also, some people are born with a congenital weakness of an artery in the brain. Over the years, as this vulnerable vessel is subjected to blood flow, especially under high pressure, it bulges more and more until it becomes a little sac called an aneurysm. An aneurysm usually does not produce any symptoms until it suddenly bursts, which is why it's been likened to a "time bomb." If you're lucky, the aneurysm may leak for a period of hours or even days instead of bursting, allowing enough time for it to be corrected surgically. (The rupture of such an aneurysm was the cause of the stroke that felled Ambassador Harriman in France in 1997. While swimming, she suddenly complained of a very severe headache, and, within minutes, lapsed into a coma from which she never recovered.)

Another congenital vascular abnormality called an arteriovenous malformation (AVM) can also cause a hemorrhagic stroke. An AVM is a cluster of abnormal blood vessels inside the brain. Unlike an aneurysm, an AVM can produce a variety of chronic symptoms such as severe headaches, seizures, and other neurological problems before it ruptures. Cerebral aneurysms and AVMs can be treated very effectively with lasers if diagnosed in time.

Regardless of its cause (thrombosis, a traveling blood clot, or a hemorrhage), the final outcome of any stroke depends on the size and the location of the blood vessel involved. If the artery is a very small one, the area of brain damaged is also small, and recovery is usually early and often complete. The larger the vessel, the more serious the symptoms and the greater the likelihood of permanent disability or death.

Diagnosing a Stroke

When your symptoms suggest a stroke, your doctor will forgo the less targeted aspects of the evaluation and focus on the neurological findings: tapping you with a little hammer, testing your muscle strength and speech, shining lights into your eyes, pricking your skin with needles or stroking it with a wisp of cotton to check sensation, listening to your speech and testing your coordination, and so on. The first decision to be made is whether or not this is a stroke. If it is, then the next question is critical: Is it due to a bleed or a blockage? If it's a thrombosis or a traveling blood clot, you will need an anticoagulant to thin your blood. But if it's a brain hemorrhage, an anticoagulant will promote bleeding and be life-threatening. This distinction usually requires the special tests described below. The right treatment can save your life; the wrong one can end it.

After the physical exam, the most important diagnostic procedure is usually the *CT (computerized tomography) scan*. Visualizing the brain in this way distinguishes a blockage from a bleed.

An *MRI (magnetic resonance imaging)* may also be done. This provides additional information as to what's actually going on in the brain—especially with regard to the precise location of the damaged area, and its size. Because it's so sensitive, the MRI is particularly useful when a small artery is involved. There is no exposure to radiation from an MRI.

MRA (magnetic resonance angiography) is a newer imaging technique that provides a view of the blood vessels themselves. It pinpoints the location of the diseased artery, yields additional information about the state of the cerebral circulation, and indicates whether or not there is a good backup or collateral circulation that can eventually take over from the diseased artery. The MRA has reduced the need to perform invasive angiograms (see below).

As I explained earlier, a stroke can result also from disease of the carotid arteries outside the brain. *Carotid duplex scanning* is a noninvasive technique that records sound waves from these vessels and indicates whether or not they are obstructed, and to what extent.

Transcranial Doppler (TCD) is another noninvasive tool. A small probe placed against the skull measures blood flow within the artery below it. Because it's portable, it can be used at the bedside to monitor the progress of a stroke and evaluate the effectiveness of therapy. A transcranial Doppler is also useful in distinguishing between a bleed and a clot, so if a CT scan is not immediately available, the TCD can be used instead.

Positron emission tomography (PET) is being used more and more these days. This technique assesses the brain's metabolism and reflects how well tissues in various parts of the brain are working after being deprived of blood. Sometimes, even after a blockage, areas of the brain assumed to have been destroyed turn out to have some function left.

Xenon CT scanning and *radionuclide SPECT scanning* are additional methods of measuring blood flow within the brain; the former uses xenon, an inert gas; the latter employs the radionuclide technetium 99.

Cerebral angiography (angiogram), though invasive, is not a high-risk procedure. It is normally the method of last resort to identify a vascular problem within the brain. Contrast dye is injected into a large artery, usually the femoral at the groin, whence it makes its way up to the brain. This technique, similar to coronary arteriography for the heart, costs about $7,000, compared to several hundred dollars for a carotid duplex or transcranial sonogram and $3,000 for an MRA. Most neurosurgeons are now willing to operate on the basis of the carotid duplex or MRI findings alone. Generally speaking, angiograms are only performed when there is a discrepancy between the findings in these two noninvasive tests.

Risk Factors for Stroke

The various mechanisms that can cause a stroke usually have several risk factors in common. These include:

- **Age:** Everything else being equal, your risk of a stroke doubles every ten years after age fifty-five.
- **High blood pressure,** untreated and of long stand-

ing, promotes and accelerates hardening of the arteries and is probably the most important controllable risk factor for stroke. Incessant pounding of the high pressure within the artery predisposes it to rupture.

• **Heart disease** and stroke go hand in hand. There are fewer heart attacks these days because of a better understanding of its causes, its prevention, and its management. (See Chapter 6.)

• **Cigarette smoking** is responsible for half the stroke deaths among Americans ages thirty-five to sixty-four, and for one in eight stroke deaths over the age of sixty-five. It is the major cause of the narrowing of the carotid artery in the neck. The nicotine, carbon monoxide, tars, resins, and other ingredients in tobacco promote the development of arteriosclerosis and cause spasm that can lead to arterial obstruction and stroke. In women, cigarettes are especially deadly when combined with oral contraceptives.

• **Abnormal blood fats:** High cholesterol, elevated triglyceride, low HDL, and raised LDL all promote the process of arteriosclerosis and thus predispose to stroke.

• **Folic acid deficiency:** If you lack a B vitamin called folic acid in your diet, an amino acid called homocysteine builds up in your blood. Homocysteine damages arteries, leads to arteriosclerosis, and may account for as many as 30 to 40 percent of all heart attacks and strokes. Most doctors still do not measure homocysteine levels in the blood nearly as often as they do cholesterol levels, but I predict that will change. I do so almost routinely in my own practice, and recommend a 400-microgram supplement of folic acid to all my adult patients, male and female.

• **Diabetes:** A high blood sugar, especially when associated with elevated blood pressure, doubles your stroke risk.

• **Transient ischemic attacks:** A TIA leaves no permanent effects, but if you've had one, you are at ten times the risk for developing a stroke in the future. So it's critical, once you've had a warning TIA, to institute the measures described below to prevent their recurrence.

• **Atrial fibrillation:** I have described earlier how and why *atrial fibrillation* causes strokes.

• **"Thick" blood:** When you have too many red blood cells, your blood is thick, clots more easily, and predisposes you to a stroke. Such an increase in the number of red blood cells can simply result from living at high altitude (the body compensates for the decreased amount of oxygen available by making more blood cells to carry whatever amount there is), or it can be due to a disorder of the bone marrow (polycythemia).

• **Sleep apnea,** characterized by snoring and irregular breathing accompanied by the rhythmic absence of respiration for a few seconds, is associated with a higher risk of stroke.

• **Obesity** is an important contributing factor to stroke, especially in women. The Nurses' Health study in Boston has, over the years, produced a great deal of interesting data in many different areas of health maintenance and disease prevention. One recent analysis revealed that women who are obese or who have gained more than forty-four pounds since the age of eighteen are 2 1/2 times more likely to suffer a thrombosis (not a hemorrhage) in the brain than are women who are lean and who have not gained a lot of weight.

• **Quick movement of the neck:** Here's one risk factor I'll bet you never thought of. No matter how old, or young, you are, a quick jerk of the neck can cause a stroke. In my most recent book, the one on alternative medicine, I cautioned against letting a chiropractor or anyone else manipulate your neck. A few days ago I received a call from a lawyer asking me to document this statement. Her client, a thirty-four-year-old woman with neck pain, ended up a quadriplegic after being treated by a chiropractor. I referred her to the journal *Neurology*, which reported that among some 180 neurologists surveyed, fifty-one stated that they had witnessed fifty-six strokes resulting from a tear in the carotid artery in the neck following a quick twist of the neck. My own chiropractor relieves my lower back pain, but I never let him go near my neck. Even your hairdresser can do you in! When you extend your neck over the basin while your hair is being washed, you can become dizzy and experience blurred vision. And although none of my own patients have had serious consequences from doing so, there have been case reports of paralysis resulting from damage to the vertebral artery, a major vessel going to the brain in the back of the neck, from such hyperextension in beauty salons.

• **There is a not-so-rare autoimmune disorder called temporal or giant cell arteritis** that affects older people—the mean age is about seventy, and the incidence increases with age. Arteries in the temple and scalp become inflamed, swollen, and tender to the touch, causing severe headaches and visual disturbances. You not only feel sick, feverish, and depressed, but these symptoms can also lead to a stroke. Fortunately, once the diagnosis of temporal arteritis is established by a biopsy of the inflamed artery, it can be successfully treated with steroid hormones, and the threat of stroke is removed.

• **Oral contraceptives:** The older ones that were available in the 1970s and 1980s did cause strokes, but the risk from newer formulations that contain less than 50 micrograms of estrogen is negligible. However, the reduced estrogen content won't help you much if you're a cigarette smoker. In my own practice, I also recommend other contraceptive techniques to women who have high blood pressure. Whether the estrogen content of the pill is high or low, we're still talking about only three or four strokes in every 100,000 users, a really rare event.

• **Sedentary lifestyle:** Physical inactivity is a risk factor for arteriosclerosis and so increases the chance of a stroke.

• **Male sex:** Here's one you can't do anything about. After the age of sixty-five, men have a 19 percent greater risk for stroke than do women, and that vulnerability is even greater earlier in life.

• **Race:** Americans of African, Mexican, Cuban, Asian, and Puerto Rican descent are more vulnerable to brain attacks than are Caucasians. You can't do anything about your heritage, but if you fall into any of these racial categories, it's especially important for you to control whatever risk factors you can identify. Blacks particularly are vulnerable because high blood pressure is so common and severe among them.

• **Where you live:** The southeastern United States is called the "stroke belt." I'm not sure why residents in this area of the country have so many brain attacks, but I suspect that diet is the main culprit. If you live in those parts, I'm not suggesting that you pack up and move. However, watch your salt and fat intake, and add plenty of fruits and vegetables to your diet.

• **Too much booze:** Binge drinking can set you up for a stroke, especially if you have other risk factors. More than two drinks a day raises blood pressure and is statistically associated with an increased incidence of brain attacks, as is drug abuse, especially using cocaine.

• **A family history of stroke** is not, in itself, a risk factor. If your parents, siblings, or other close blood relatives had a stroke, you're not more likely to suffer one unless you ignore one or more of the risk factors listed above.

How to Prevent a Stroke

To reduce your chances of getting a stroke, start thinking about prevention while you're still young. Here are some specifics:

• **Regular medical checkups** identify the risk factors to which you may be vulnerable. During a routine physical your doctor examines you, weighs you, measures your blood pressure, checks your cholesterol and related blood lipids, sugar and other blood chemistries, and reviews your lifestyle and habits (such as smoking or exercise). He or she can then recommend whatever steps need to be taken. I frequently detect the irregular rhythm (atrial fibrillation) that can lead to blood clots traveling to the brain in patients who are completely unaware of having it.

• **Normalizing high blood pressure:** This is the single most important step you can take, at any age, to prevent stroke. But you must keep checking your pressure on an ongoing basis. A normal reading when you're forty-five years old is no guarantee that it will remain so when you're forty-six.

Many people are under the impression that as long as the bottom blood pressure number, the diastolic, is normal, a high systolic reading is not important. That's a serious error. *Any* blood pressure elevation, systolic or diastolic, is a major risk factor for stroke. What's a normal reading? We used to consider anything below 140/90 acceptable. We now know that the lower the reading, the better, so you should aim for somewhere in the neighborhood of 110–120/70–80. I'm often asked by patients whether it's "still important" to lower their pressure in later years. Of course it is! Hypertension can lead to stroke at any age. You're never too old to have a normal pressure.

There are several steps to normalizing an elevated pressure. If you're overweight, just shedding enough pounds may do it; regular exercise also helps keep pressure in check; a low-salt diet works for some people, although many cases of hypertension are not salt-dependent.

I advise all my hypertensive patients, especially those over sixty-five, to reduce the amount of salt in their diet to less than 2,000 milligrams a day (a level teaspoon of salt contains about 2,400 milligrams). The average daily consumption in this country is closer to 9 to 10 grams a day. Here are some other pertinent facts:

Fresh food usually contains the least amount of salt. The main problem is the 75 percent of dietary salt that's hidden in processed foods such as hot dogs, canned foods, processed meats, and frozen pizza. Removing the saltshaker from your table can reduce your salt intake by 10 percent. Use only enough salt in the cooking to give your food the taste you want.

About 15 percent of your salt intake is from obviously salty foods such as schmaltz or pickled herring. That's easy enough to give up if you have the willpower.

Eating out also presents problems. I love Chinese food, so imagine my dismay when I learned that an order of fried rice in my favorite restaurant contains almost 3,000 milligrams of salt, while a fried seafood platter has almost 5,000.

Read the labels on all packaged foods. See how much sodium a product contains in any form—disodium phosphate, monosodium glutamate, sodium nitrate, and others.

Perhaps even more important than sodium restriction

is a diet rich in fruits and vegetables. The calcium and potassium they contain lower blood pressure independently of any other steps you take.

If your pressure is elevated, chances are you will eventually need medication. There is a widespread belief that all drugs used to control high blood pressure can destroy your libido and cause other unpleasant side effects. Not so. The newer agents, especially when used in combination and in small amounts, can almost always effectively lower blood pressure without intolerable side effects. A word of caution, however: Some of these agents are very potent. If you're over sixty and have no other health problems, start with a diuretic. Water pills are the least expensive of all the medications available and have few side effects. Too many doctors rush into the more sophisticated and costly agents before giving diuretics a try. The main exceptions to the "diuretic-first" suggestion is the presence of gout (which diuretics can aggravate), certain kinds of kidney disease, and dehydration. Whatever drug you take, start with the smallest dose. A sharp, sudden drop in blood pressure can cause a stroke too.

• **Preventive carotid artery surgery (endarterectomy):** Suppose that in the course of a routine examination, your doctor listens to the arteries in your neck and hears a "bruit." This suggests that the caliber of the underlying artery is narrowed by an arteriosclerotic plaque. Even if you have no symptoms, that finding should be evaluated by the carotid duplex test described earlier. If you're found to have a significant blockage, say 60 percent or more, and you have neurological symptoms attributable to it, the plaque should be removed. But what should you do if you have a plaque and feel perfectly well? Should you simply stay on aspirin or other anticoagulants? Should the plaque be removed? After years of controversy, the medical profession has finally agreed that even when these blockages are not causing any symptoms they should usually be removed if the obstruction is 60 to 70 percent or greater. As a result of this consensus, there were more than 100,000 such procedures done in 1996 as compared to 68,000 only six years earlier.

Surgery is no longer the only option. The blocked artery can often be ballooned open (angioplastied) just like the coronary arteries, and even stented, in which case rigid props are inserted into the diseased artery (with or without prior angioplasty) to keep it open. However, this latter procedure is still in the early stages of development and complication rates are on the high side.

• **The right diet** goes a long way toward preventing strokes. That's news to the 82 percent of Americans polled in 1995 who had no idea that lowering cholesterol helps prevent stroke as well as heart attacks. The obvious culprit is fat, especially saturated animal fat and cholesterol. So substitute skim milk, low-fat cheeses, and other low-fat dairy products for whole milk, cheese, and cream. Concentrate on a diet rich in fruits and vegetables, fish (at least two servings a week), pasta, rice, bread, and cereal. In one study, women who ate just one carrot a day for several years had 68 percent fewer strokes; onions help, too, by thinning the blood, and so does garlic; spinach also lowers the risk of stroke (and heart disease too). Limit yourself to three egg yolks a week. Eat less red meat, none of it with visible fat. That means buying lean cuts, trimming off any fat you can see, and removing the skin from poultry before cooking it. And get into the habit of baking, steaming, roasting, or broiling your food rather than frying it.

The FDA has recently approved the use of the statin drugs that lower cholesterol to prevent stroke and transient ischemic attacks, even when levels are in the so-called normal range. There is evidence that these medications can cut the incidence of stroke by at least 30 percent in persons with heart disease, and by 14 percent in healthy individuals. However, anything that reduces the risk of arteriosclerosis—exercise, maintaining ideal body weight, a proper diet—will also decrease the risk of stroke. Recent research suggests that alpha-linoleic acid, an ingredient of canola oil, is also helpful.

In Japan, where the consumption of fat has been increasing over the years, the stroke rate (always notoriously high in that country) has actually dropped. But here's the rub: During this same period, the number of heart attacks has increased. This suggests that heart attacks and strokes may have different causative mechanisms. However, these observations are preliminary. My advice is still to eschew a high-fat diet.

• **Thinning the blood (anticoagulants) when necessary:** If you have atrial fibrillation, the irregular rhythm described earlier, you are at great risk for developing a stroke. That's because in the presence of the irregular rhythm, little clots can form within the heart. When one of them is squeezed out, it can travel to the brain and obstruct an artery. The only way to reduce the chances of that happening is to "thin" the blood, and the best medication for that purpose is an anticoagulant called warfarin (Coumadin). Believe it or not, warfarin is a rat poison. When the animal eats enough of it, it bleeds to death. But you won't, because when you're taking Coumadin your blood is checked at regular intervals to make sure it's like Goldilocks's porridge—not too thick and not too thin, but just right.

Coumadin therapy has its drawbacks. For instance, you need a blood test every three or four weeks to regulate the dose; there is the danger of an internal hemorrhage if you take too much; and if you're in an accident or need immediate surgery, you may have a bleeding problem. But on balance, doctors agree that most fibrillators should be taking Coumadin. Unfortunately, only one-fourth of those who need the drug currently receive it. Naturally, if you have a bleeding ulcer or some other condition that militates against your taking anticoagulants, you mustn't do so.

In an attempt to avoid the inconvenience and risks of Coumadin, aspirin was carefully studied to see whether it could do as good a job at preventing traveling clots. The conclusion? It's better than no blood thinning at all, and you should take it if you can't tolerate Coumadin, but it's not as effective.

Are you one of the 77 percent of people who don't know that *quitting smoking* will reduce your stroke risk within two to five years after you kick the habit? There are immediate benefits too. Every time you inhale tobacco smoke, it causes spasm of arteries of every size throughout the body, including the brain. If you've already got some little plaques there, and most adults do, then the additional spasm insult can cause at least a TIA or ministroke.

• **Controlling sugar levels in diabetics** is an important preventive measure against stroke. Chronically elevated blood sugar predisposes virtually every organ in the body, including the brain, to vascular disease.

• **Getting enough folic acid** is an important step in preventing at least 15 percent, and possibly even more, of all strokes. Make sure your diet includes at least 400 micrograms of this vitamin. That's the amount found in most multivitamin preparations. It will also protect against heart disease, and if you happen to be pregnant, against birth defects too.

Most doctors agree that hormone replacement therapy after menopause lowers the incidence of heart disease and modifies the course of Alzheimer's, too. You'd expect that it would have the same beneficial effect on stroke, but apparently, according to the most recent research reports, it does not.

Treating a Stroke: 911

The number to remember is 911. The key word in the treatment of a stroke is *time*. When someone has a stroke in this country, the average interval between the onset of symptoms and the examination by a doctor is anywhere from six to twenty-four hours! In one large study, less than half of the stroke patients consulted a physician within twenty-four hours, and one-third sought no help for more than two days! Yet the new, life-saving drugs that can dissolve the clot that's causing the stroke must be administered within three hours after the onset of symptoms. So if you wait for any reason—because you're denying what you suspect may be true and hope it will go away, or you're not sure what your symptoms mean but are an optimist and are confident that everything's going to be fine, or you think there's nothing to do anyway because if it is a stroke, your number is up, or any other ridiculous excuse people make—you'll miss the boat. *If you think you may be having a stroke, take an aspirin immediately, and then get to the nearest hospital emergency room.*

When you arrive, things will move fast. The triage nurse knows not to keep you waiting. An intravenous will be started immediately. At first it will deliver only some sugar and water into your veins just to keep them open in the event that you need medication. Next comes the oxygen ritual, delivered through little prongs inserted into your nostrils. You'll then have a neurologically focused physical. This is no time for elaborate history taking; it's too late for questions like "What did your great-uncle die of, and how old was he?" Speed is of the essence. If the neurological exam indicates a stroke, you will immediately have a CT scan to determine whether it's due to a bleed or a blockage.

If you're found to have a clot, the drug that can help dissolve it is called *t-PA*. It's usually given by vein, although more recently doctors have been injecting it into an artery to see if the results can be even further improved. No matter how it is administered, you must receive t-PA within three hours after the onset of your symptoms. This therapy reduces the chance of residual paralysis by 50 percent. Its major risk is bleeding within the brain when you receive too much.

If the CT scan reveals evidence of a bleed and not a clot, your blood pressure will be monitored and kept at normal levels, and your heart function will be supported. Of course, there is the inevitable oxygen, and drugs to reduce swelling in the injured area of the brain may be administered. The possibility of surgery to correct the cause of the bleed will be considered if it's due to a ruptured arterio-venous malformation or cerebral aneurysm. These events used to be uniformly fatal. However, these days, if you're in the right place at the right time, the brain hemorrhage they cause can sometimes be surgically corrected by *stereotactic microsurgery*. This is a dramatic new procedure that uses sophisticated computer technology and geometric principles to locate the precise point of bleeding in the brain. Delicate instruments and microscope-enhanced methods can repair the bleeding site without harming nearby healthy brain tissue. A variation of such surgery, *stereotactic radiosurgery*, uses radiation. The bleeding site is localized in the same way but instead of an operation, a beam of radiation pinpointed at the area coagulates the leaking vessel. During both the surgical and radiation treatment of these cerebral hemorrhages, the patient's body is usually cooled, or a cardiopulmonary bypass machine is used, to prevent further damage. Some centers also introduce a tiny catheter into the arterial circulation and use a *superglue* to block off the bleeding site.

If a clot caused your stroke but you were too late for t-PA, all is not lost. You may be given another anticoagulant called *low-molecular-weight heparin* (LMWH). Six months after a stroke, patients who receive this drug have a 31 percent better result than patients who are not so treated.

And don't forget *aspirin*! You should have taken one the moment you suspected a stroke. We used to hold off on the aspirin until stroke patients were ready for discharge from the hospital, but we now know that it's important in treating the acute stage of stroke.

To help prevent a second stroke, most doctors will have you continue taking aspirin indefinitely. The enteric-coated "baby dose" of 81 milligrams is widely used to prevent heart attacks, but after a stroke you're better off taking at least one or more regular-strength (325-milligram) aspirin tablets.

If you can't tolerate aspirin, there's another "blood-thinner," an antiplatelet agent called clopidogrel (Plavix). I was impressed with the results of a recent landmark trial, the largest clinical trial ever conducted on any medicine in development. Clopidogrel was found to prevent a third of strokes, heart attacks, or vascular deaths in patients at risk because of an earlier attack. By comparison, aspirin reduced the occurrence rate by 25 percent. This study also revealed that clopidogrel, which works on the platelets to prevent clotting much like aspirin does, is also just as safe. But, as with aspirin, don't take Plavix if you have a bleeding problem.

The drug of last resort in my practice is Ticlid, even though it's effective. I try to avoid it because it can occasionally cause a potentially fatal blood disorder called thrombotic thrombocytopenic purpura within four weeks after therapy is begun. There is mass destruction of the blood platelets, kidney failure, and neurological changes. These complications, though not common, are most apt to occur in patients over sixty years of age.

If a stroke is due to thrombosis of a large artery, your doctor may elect to treat you with *Coumadin* rather than with aspirin, Plavix, or Ticlid at least for the first few weeks or months.

A recent approach to the treatment of acute stroke now being investigated is the "neuroprotective" agents. The one that's received the most publicity to date is a synthetic steroid called *pregnanolone hemisuccinate (Selfotel)*. When brain cells (neurons) die, they release a substance called glutamate. As more and more glutamate is produced, it spreads within the brain, attacks healthy neurons, and kills them, too. Selfotel prevents release of this harmful chemical.

There's one treatment for a stroke, regardless of whether it's due to a bleed or a clot, that isn't used as much as it should be. Researchers in the Department of Neurology at the Boston University School of Medicine reported that some patients who were treated with *acupuncture* after a stroke (not necessarily within the three hours required for t-PA, but the sooner the better) had a significant reduction in the late incidence of paralysis. I'm not quite sure how acupuncture works in this situation. Perhaps it causes the brain to release certain hormones that dilate the blood vessels around the diseased area, or it may create new electrical pathways for nerve impulses to travel. Since there is no downside to using acupuncture (assuming that the needles are clean and disposable), I know I'd ask for this treatment if I ever had a stroke, in addition to all the other conventional therapy.

After the Stroke

Although strokes do not result in permanent disability as often as they once did, they still cripple a large number of people.

The most common complications are paralysis or weakness of one side or part of the body, the inability to speak and understand, learning problems, impaired memory, loss of motor skills, and behavioral and emotional changes.

There has been considerable progress in poststroke rehabilitation in the past few years. Stroke victims with residual paralysis are no longer incarcerated in some facility or left at home and forgotten. Rehabilitation departments **are able** to coordinate the skills of a variety of health-care experts—doctors, physical and occupational therapists, nurses, social workers, speech and language therapists, conventional and alternative medicine professionals—who can help patients in many ways. I have seen countless stroke victims who were unable to dress themselves, get out of a chair, feed themselves, or perform other basic functions dramatically improve after treatment by these dedicated specialists. Muscle strength, eye-hand coordination, and the skills needed to bathe and even cook for themselves can often be restored. The goal of every such program should be maximum independence and the return, to an active and productive life.

The rehabilitation process begins while you're still in the hospital. After you leave, you must be connected with the right team in the right place—at home or at some other convenient setting. In the hospital where I work, stroke survivors with residual impairments are usually discharged to an affiliated convalescent or chronic care facility where skilled personnel can assess their specific problems and work intensively to correct them. The patient returns home for ongoing physiotherapy provided by community agencies only after maximum improvement has been attained.

What to Remember about Stroke

1. A stroke is a brain attack. It is to the brain what a heart attack is to the heart.

2. There are two main types of stroke: those that result from the obstruction of blood flow to the brain because an artery supplying some portion of it is obstructed, and those that occur because of a hemorrhage within the brain, usually due to the bursting of a blood vessel.

3. Treatment of stroke depends on whether it was caused by a blockage or a bleed. This information is best and most quickly obtained by means of a CT scan of the brain.

4. Symptoms of a stroke come on suddenly. The main ones are sudden weakness, numbness, or paralysis of the face, arm, or leg (especially on one side of the body); loss of speech, or trouble with speaking or with understanding language; sudden loss of vision, particularly in one eye; sudden severe headache of unknown cause; unexplained dizziness; loss of balance or coordination.

5. A stroke is a prime medical emergency. If you suspect you're having one, get to a hospital immediately. The most important measures that can prevent permanent damage to the brain must be started within three hours after the onset of symptoms.

6. There are many risk factors for stroke, the most important of which are high blood pressure, diabetes, and heart disease and all the factors that predispose to it such as high cholesterol, being overweight, and physical inactivity. Controlling them can effectively lower the risk of stroke.

7. Atrial fibrillation, an irregular rhythm, is a major cause of stroke whose risk can be reduced by thinning the blood with the drug warfarin and, somewhat less effectively, by aspirin.

8. Arteriosclerotic plaques can narrow the carotid arteries in the neck without causing any symptoms. Your doctor can detect these when he or she listens to the neck area with a stethoscope. If there is a 60 percent or greater obstruction to blood flow, removing the plaques can prevent a stroke.

9. A clot-dissolving chemical, t-PA, when injected into a vein or artery within three hours of a stroke, can reduce the risk of long-term disability.

10. Once you've had a stroke, taking aspirin or other anticoagulants indefinitely can reduce the risk of recurrence.

11. Dedicated, skilled rehabilitation programs can improve residual paralysis and other stroke complications.

16

DIMINISHED TASTE AND SMELL

A Tasteless Chapter!

I don't know why I relive so many of my childhood memories while writing this book on aging. Each topic brings back different and indelible recollections. In preparing this chapter on the decreased perception of taste and smell, I recall vividly the many festive dinners at our home when my parents, aunts, uncles, and their close friends ate, drank, and made merry. Mostly, however, they ate. I couldn't understand at the time why they all added so much sugar, salt, pepper, and other condiments to every dish and beverage—even the chicken soup, my mother's specialty. I can still recall its exquisite aroma as she brought it to the table, steaming. It was heavenly. The taste was divine—just right. Yet to my amazement, every single guest added lots and lots of salt. And they dropped innumerable cubes or heaping teaspoons of sugar into their tea—any tea: green, black, jasmine, or mint. They apparently also felt that even the meat, already koshered with lots of salt, needed much more taste, dousing it with additional salt, and pepper too. Regardless of what they ate or drank, and often without even first tasting it, my elderly relatives and their friends always added some spice, condiment, or flavor enhancer to virtually every dish.

Now you'd think my mother would be offended by the gross tampering with her dishes. But she was not—not in the least. What's more, she too added extra salt and pepper to every dish she prepared—even to her absolutely perfect chicken soup!

My wife was very young when we were married. One of the first things I requested of her after our honeymoon was that she ask my mother for that chicken soup recipe. She did, and we dined deliciously on it almost forever after. I say almost because a few years ago, after some thirty-five years of marriage, my wife seemed to be losing her touch not only for making my mother's soup, but for preparing other dishes as well. They all suddenly needed salt, pepper, and other condiments. She insisted she was following all the old recipes to a T; I even supervised the preparation of the soup myself. So why, after all these years, did it now need salt?

Older people (myself included) enhance the flavor of everything they consume because of their decreased acuity of taste and smell. The next time you're at a dinner party, look around and see who uses the salt and pepper shakers most. Chances are it's the older diners. It has been calculated that on the average, they add eleven times as much salt, and three times the amount of sugar, to their food as do younger people.

More than 2 million Americans have some disorder of

taste and/or smell perception, and most of them are older. They pay over 200,000 medical visits every year to have their impaired sense of taste treated. Countless others probably don't bother to complain—they just add salt to everything they eat.

Taste and smell gradually begin to decline after age thirty. The change is subtle for the first few years, but as you approach sixty, you are usually aware of a decrease in the acuity of your senses of taste and smell. By the time you're seventy (later, and to a lesser extent, in women) your food doesn't taste the same anymore. You wonder why so many of your favorite chefs (and husbands and wives) have lost their touch. It's not only the taste of the food; the aroma is also apt to be less powerful.

Loss of smell can be selective, so that you may perceive some odors and not others. I recently advised my wife (who is much, much younger than I) to try a very comprehensive multivitamin formula rich in vitamin B complex She reminded me that the odor of vitamin B turns her stomach. "These won't," I assured her. "They're odorless. See, they don't have any smell," I said, after I opened the bottle and held them to my nose. I smelled nothing—but she gagged!

Flavor is what makes eating and drinking such a pleasure. It's defined as the interaction of aroma, taste, texture, appearance, temperature, and "spiciness." (The Kellogg's people think that sound is important too; hence, the "Snap Crackle Pop" of their Rice Krispies.)

How We Taste and Smell

Taste and smell are dependent on at least three different but mutually interacting chemosenses. A small patch of tissue high up in the nose, called the olfactory membrane, makes it possible for us to perceive and identify odors. The olfactory membrane consists of 100 million receptors containing 10,000 *different* kinds of cells. If they were all identical, everything would smell the same. It's their variability that permits us to distinguish one aroma from another. (To Surrey, my German shepherd, 100 million is a paltry number. She has 1 billion such cells, which is why, from three rooms away, she knows when I've unwrapped a chocolate bar.) When an odor reaches these nasal receptors, they process it and send it to the olfactory (smell) nerve for transmission to the brain.

Taste involves a different mechanism. When saliva dissolves your food, the molecules that are released travel to the 9,000 cells that make up the taste buds in the mouth and throat. There are 100 cells per bud, many of which are visible as little bumps scattered about the tongue. These buds detect and identify four basic tastes: sweet and salty (perceived mainly on the front of the tongue), sour (on the sides), and bitter (mostly in the back). This information is transmitted to the brain by special nerve cells.

There is yet a third mechanism, called common chemical sense, that helps us recognize the irritating properties of substances in the mouth and odors in the nose. It's this sense that conveys the heat of chili peppers, the coolness of menthol, and the sting of ammonia. It consists of thousands of nerve endings on the moist surfaces of the eyes, mouth, nose, and throat. A separate set of nerves conveys this information to the brain.

There are different degrees of impairment of taste and smell. You may lose your sense of smell completely (anosmia) or only partially (hyposmia); taste loss can be total (ageusia) or limited (hypogeusia). There are some variations on this theme; parosmia refers to phantom smells, the perception of odors that don't really exist. Someone with parosmia is convinced that everyone around him or her stinks. Its counterpart in taste is dysgeusia, when everything consumed tastes bad.

All our "chemosenses" are important and enhance each other to maximize our appreciation of food, and nothing tastes quite the same if any one of them breaks down. If your sense of smell is impaired, your enjoyment of food is diminished. In fact, an intact "smelling sense" accounts for 75 percent of the flavor you perceive. If you need to be convinced of that, try holding your nose and closing your eyes. Have someone put some food in your mouth. Chances are you won't be able to tell a turnip from an apple, or detect the flavor of chocolate. Nor will you fully savor coffee. (The flavors of chocolate and coffee, like many other substances, are largely sensed by their aroma.) If you lose your sense of smell, you may not be able to taste what you're eating even if your taste buds are intact.

Confirming the Diagnosis

To evaluate your loss of taste or smell, your doctor will first perform some simple tests. For example, can you tell if there is sugar in your coffee? He or she may apply different chemicals to specific parts of your tongue for you to identify (the "sip, spit, and rinse" test). There is also the "scratch and sniff" test, in which you scratch a piece of paper pretreated with a variety of chemicals. You then sniff, and try to identify the various odors that are released. The best agents for evaluating smell are vanilla, coffee, and cloves. In addition to such simple determinations, you will also need a thorough examination of your mouth and nose, a neurological evaluation, and possibly a CT scan or MRI of the head.

Changes That Occur with Aging

As we get older, taste becomes less acute for several reasons. Because we produce less saliva, the molecules in our food are not transported as efficiently to the taste buds. And the taste buds themselves are reduced in size and number. By the time you're seventy, you have half the number of taste buds you had when you were twenty. The buds at the front of the tongue, which detect sweetness and salt, are the first to go; those in the back and on the sides of the tongue, for bitter and sour, are affected later. So by age seventy, you're apt to detect fewer sweet and salty flavors, and more bitter or sour tastes.

Even more important than these changes in the mouth is the decrease in the number of smell receptors in the nose. We never completely lose taste and smell as we grow older because these smell receptor cells are replaced as they are damaged or die. No other cells in the nervous system have this capability. Significant symptoms develop only when these cells are lost more rapidly than they're replaced.

Causes of Loss of Taste and Smell Other than Aging

• **Viral infections** such as the flu or a bad cold can kill some smell and taste receptors. The older you are, the longer it takes for these senses to return, but the damage is sometimes permanent.

• **Trauma to the head** (a blow or injury of some kind, even one so trivial you may not even remember it) can affect taste and smell.

• **Congestion due to any cause,** ranging from the common cold to hay fever or other nasal allergies that leave you stuffed up, will affect smell and taste.

• **Nasal polyps** can prevent air from reaching the tissues high up in the nose that detect aromas. Chronic sinusitis, or an operation on the nose or sinuses, can sometimes impair the sense of smell. Smell receptors can be damaged by chronic exposure to gasoline, benzene, paint thinner, other organic solvents, certain chemicals such as chlorine and mercury, metal and wood dusts, and insecticides.

- **Pollution,** the most important source of which is tobacco, has an impact on smell and taste. If you quit smoking now, these senses can be restored but it may take years.
- **Infections** such as shingles or Bell's palsy, or radiation therapy to the facial area, can damage the nerves that transmit the taste and smell signals to the brain.
- **A variety of neurological disorders,** including brain tumors, Parkinson's disease, Alzheimer's, and stroke, can all impair taste and smell.
- **Diabetes, low thyroid function, and hepatitis** can affect these senses.
- **Dryness of the mouth** due to any cause decreases taste perception. Common causes of a dry mouth include heavy pipe smoking, the aging process (because of a decreased production of saliva), and Sjögren's syndrome, an autoimmune disorder most commonly seen in postmenopausal women.
- **Deficiency of vitamin B$_{12}$ (pernicious anemia),** as well as a lack of zinc, copper, and vitamin A, in the diet can all affect taste and smell.
- **Medications are common culprits.** These include captopril (a drug commonly used to treat high blood pressure), such anti-cancer agents as cisplatin, vinblastine, and vincristine, chronic use of nasal-decongestant nose drops and sprays, amphetamines, lithium (used in the treatment of manic-depression), griseofulvin (the antifungal agent), penicillamine (for the treatment of rheumatoid arthritis), and various tranquilizers.

So if you find that your food no longer tastes like it

should or you don't perceive aromas as well as you once did, let your doctor know. It's not necessarily your age; he or she may recommend something as simple as an antihistamine to treat your allergy or suggest you use a vaporizer or humidifier. An offending medication, once identified, can be changed or withdrawn; a physical blockage in your nose can be surgically corrected. Some doctors prescribe zinc supplements when a viral infection is the cause of your problem (15 milligrams a day combined with vitamin C). I have never been convinced that this therapy works, except in cases of obvious zinc deficiency, but it's worth a try. Steroid therapy may also help. Who knows? You may even be persuaded to stop smoking.

As a rule, if you've had these symptoms for six months or longer, the chance of them ever clearing up is remote, regardless of what you do.

It's important to try to add to the enjoyment of your food so that you don't become depressed or malnourished. If your sense of smell or taste is impaired, eat lots of hot, highly seasoned foods and use potent condiments and concentrated essences that don't irritate the stomach. Such crunchy foods as nuts, croutons, or water chestnuts will also enhance your enjoyment of food. Combining hot and cold temperatures in the same dish (sour cream on a hot potato or, for the more affluent, caviar on a blini) may make it more interesting. And be sure to take multivitamin supplements to compensate for any nutritional deficiencies in your diet.

Other Important Steps to Take

Whatever the cause of your impaired taste and smell, you must take the following steps to protect yourself since you may not be able to detect smoke, gas, and other poisonous fumes, or recognize that some dish you are about to eat is spoiled. Install audible smoke alarms in your home. If you have any gas appliances, get a gas detector. Better still, replace them with electrical equipment. If you have high blood pressure, use salt substitutes instead of salt. If you're diabetic, don't add sugar to your tea and coffee; use artificial sweeteners. Date all the food you put in your refrigerator, and be sure to store it at appropriate temperatures. Also, be sure to check the expiration date on all perishable items. Examine all food very carefully for evidence of spoiling before you eat it. Whenever possible, have someone else check your food before you prepare and eat it.

What to Remember about Taste and Smell

1. The aging process is associated with a decrease in the number of cells responsible for taste and smell.
2. Although there is no specific treatment for this disorder, many of its causes can be successfully treated. These should always be identified before you accept your symptoms as inevitable.

3. Aside from aging, the three major conditions responsible for loss of taste and smell are viral infections, head injuries, and nasal disorders.

4. If you've lost your sense of taste or smell, you are vulnerable to environmental hazards, such as smoke, gas leaks, and spoiled food. Learn how to protect yourself against these dangers.

17

TINNITUS

For Whom the Bell Tolls—
and Tolls, and Tolls

While I was making morning rounds recently, one of my patients, an elderly man with a heart rhythm problem, really lit into me. "Doc, I never want to come back to this hospital again. If I get sick, send me anywhere else, but not here. They really don't give a damn about the patients in this place." This was a devastating accusation against an institution where I have spent most of my professional life. I was shocked. Frankly, I wouldn't have been surprised if he'd complained about the food, the elevator service, or the fluctuating room temperatures, but no one had ever before suggested that my hospital "doesn't care." "What's wrong?" I asked. "What happened?"

"What happened?" he countered. "You don't know? What kind of hospital allows construction to go on all night outside the rooms of sick people—all the banging and sawing and buzzing. I didn't sleep a wink."

"What time did they stop?" I asked.

"Stop? Are you kidding? They're still at it. Just listen."

I heard nothing and looked out the window. There was no construction in sight. It turns out that the sounds that had kept this man awake were coming from within his own head. This phenomenon is called tinnitus, and in his case, it was the result of the medication, quinidine, we had given him to regularize his heart rhythm.

Some 40 million Americans, about one in every seven or eight, and a third of all people over sixty-five years of age are plagued by noise generated in their heads. Tinnitus has been described as ringing, hissing, knocking, buzzing, pounding, roaring, blowing, humming, sizzling, clanging, popping, and clicking, among others. The variety of sounds is endless.

The word *tinnitus* is derived from the Latin *tinnere*, meaning to "ring" or "tinkle"—like a bell. The sound may come and go, but often becomes permanent and an integral part of your life. You may perceive it in one ear or in both, or somewhere else in the head. It sometimes even seems to originate outside the body.

Most people with tinnitus can cope with and adjust to it, but in as many as 6 percent of cases, it seriously affects the quality of life.

William Shatner, the actor best known for his role in *Star Trek,* revealed in an interview with *People* magazine some years ago that he suffered from tinnitus. The noise in his head was so bad that at one point he didn't really care to go on living. (Interestingly, another member of his "crew," Leonard Nimoy, also had tinnitus. Since their "spaceship" never left the studio, we can't blame interplanetary travel for their symptoms.)

To give you some idea of what a tinnitus victim endures, imagine being holed up in a small apartment right beside an airport runway with jets constantly landing and taking off. The roar of the engines is there every single moment of the day and night—while you're eating, reading, thinking, making love, talking on the phone, trying to sleep, listening to music, or watching television. You're constantly enveloped in a loud roar from which there is no escape; there are no doors to shut, no earplugs to wear, nowhere to go.

Two Types of Tinnitus

Tinnitus, like fever or pain, is a symptom, not a disease. It can be subjective (only you hear the sounds), or objective (someone else can hear them too).

OBJECTIVE TINNITUS

The causes of objective tinnitus include an arthritic jaw joint that creaks when you chew, bones in the neck that make a grating sound when you turn your head, a blocked Eustachian tube in the middle ear that clicks when you swallow, repetitive contractions of the muscles in the palate in the mouth, blood throbbing as it courses through a partially obstructed carotid artery in the neck on its way to the brain, or the normal hum of blood flowing in the jugular vein.

I first heard objective tinnitus when I was a teenager. I had a sexy, beautiful girlfriend named Margie who sat at the desk next to mine at school. Whenever we went out on a date, she would tease me with "Want to hear my click?" We would then sit cheek-to-cheek, ear-to-ear, while she moved her jaw to produce an audible click. I never understood what caused it, and, frankly, I couldn't care less, but it did turn me on. To this day, I have a conditioned, very pleasant response to any clicking sound.

SUBJECTIVE TINNITUS

Subjective tinnitus, when no one but you can hear the sound, is more common than the objective variety. Subjective tinnitus can occur at any age, and has many possible causes. However, in this chapter, I focus on the tinnitus associated with aging, or as one physician put it, when "the patient is literally listening to old age sneaking up."

Tinnitus of Aging

The same mechanism that causes presbycusis (the inability to hear high tones as we get older, see Chapter 5) also accounts for tinnitus. The tiny hairs in the cochlea of the inner ear that normally convert sound vibrations into electrical energy transmitted to the brain by the auditory nerve are reduced in number and don't function normally. They begin to discharge spontaneously and send to the brain noises (impulses) that originate within the ear. Think of it as a form of internal static ignored by young, healthy hair cells in abundance, but on which they focus and magnify when they are old. These unwanted sounds are independent of hearing, so that stone-deaf persons can still be plagued by them.

Tinnitus of aging can never be cured because the reduction in number and impaired function of the hair cells is irreversible. Neither can it be prevented, although some hearing specialists believe that chronic exposure to noise over the years predisposes to both hearing loss and tinnitus later on in life.

Other Causes of Tinnitus

Before you blame the noises in your head on your age, make sure you don't have any of the following curable, treatable causes of tinnitus that can affect anyone from six to sixty-five.

• **Wax in the ear canal.** No matter how old or how young you are, before embarking on a time-consuming, costly tinnitus workup, have someone look into your ear canal. An obstructing plug of wax can not only impair your hearing, it can often cause tinnitus, too. What a relief to have the incessant sound disappear after the wax is removed. But don't poke anything, not even a Q-Tip, into your ear. If you suspect wax, ask your local druggist for a 50 percent solution of hydrogen peroxide or other wax-dissolving product (Ceruminex) that you can instill yourself. Lie down, put the solution in your ear with a dropper, and tilt your head first to one side then the other for a few minutes. After the wax has dissolved, fill a small syringe with warm water and gently rinse it out. More cases of deafness and tinnitus have been cured by removing earwax than by all other treatments combined.

• **High blood pressure** pounds relentlessly against the walls of the arteries everywhere in the body, causing them to "harden"—that is, to become arteriosclerotic. When this process also affects the tiny vessels in the inner ear, it makes them abnormally rigid, so that the blood flowing through them produces tinnitus. Reducing an elevated pressure can prevent such tinnitus or lessen its severity.

• **Prolonged bouts of high sugar** can lead to tinnitus, regardless of age. So if you're diabetic, keep your blood sugar within normal limits. If you have tinnitus of aging and are also diabetic, good sugar control may reduce the intensity of the noises in your head.

• **When arthritis** distorts and misshapes the bones in the neck, it can throw muscles in the area into spasm, causing objective and subjective tinnitus. Anything that controls or eliminates this spasm (physiotherapy, anti-inflammatory drugs) may improve tinnitus.

• **Any disease process in the brain,** such as a stroke or an infection, can cause tinnitus. There are also two kinds of tumors situated in the middle ear—acoustic neuroma and a glomus tumor—that almost invariably do so. Both these growths must be looked for whenever tinnitus develops abruptly. Their removal eliminates the symptom.

• **A blow or other injury to the head, neck, or ears,** or whiplash damage to the spine, can cause a concussion, swelling of brain tissue, or nerve injury—and tinnitus. Tinnitus following such an accident may be temporary or permanent, depending on what organ was hurt, how severely, and in what way.

• **Emotional stress** probably can't cause tinnitus, but it can make it worse. When you're tense, worried, or depressed, any symptom, including tinnitus, is magnified.

• **There are more than 200 different drugs** that can give you tinnitus, especially when taken over a long period of time or in large doses. The most frequently implicated are aspirin; quinine, which is present in tonic water and in medication to control leg cramps; quinidine, used in the treatment of certain disorders of heart rhythm; furosemide (Lasix), a widely prescribed diuretic or water pill; etharcrynic acid (Edecrin), another water pill; Talwin, a painkiller; and chloroquine, for the prevention of malaria. If you develop tinnitus while taking any of these medications, chances are they are the cause.

• **Any food allergy** can produce temporary tinnitus. Aficionados of Chinese food prepared with monosodium glutamate (MSG) are especially vulnerable. If you have tinnitus and suspect that MSG may be the cause, ask your waiter to omit it from the cooking.

• **Alcohol** can frequently cause tinnitus, particularly in the hangover phase. Once you dry out, the head noises usually disappear. If you have mild, underlying tinnitus, a hangover will make it worse.

• **Marijuana** can cause tinnitus and/or worsen existing tinnitus. If your head starts ringing after you light up, do what some famous people suggest: Don't inhale.

• **Caffeine** in coffee, tea, cola drinks, chocolate, and cocoa won't cause tinnitus—but can worsen it, especially when taken in large amounts. If you suspect that caffeine's your problem, eliminate it for about a month and see what happens.

• **Nicotine,** responsible for so many of mankind's ills, can also cause or worsen tinnitus.

• **Certain antibiotics,** such as streptomycin, neomycin, kanamycin, and gentamicin, can result in deafness by affecting the hair cells in the cochlea, and they can cause tinnitus by the same mechanism. If you're taking one of them, and tinnitus (or deafness) sets in, tell your doctor. If you absolutely need one of these drugs, there's some good news on the horizon. When researchers at the University of Michigan pretreated guinea pigs with iron-chelating drugs (they soak up extra iron in the bloodstream) these antibiotics did not cause deafness. Clinical trials of these chelating agents are now underway in humans.

• **Ménière's disease** is an ear disorder characterized by dizziness, nausea, progressive hearing loss, a feeling of fullness behind the ears—and tinnitus. Treatment, which is not very effective, consists mainly of a low-salt diet and diuretics. There are operations available for very severe cases when all else fails. Unfortunately, such surgery is akin to throwing the baby out with the bathwater because while it does eliminate the tinnitus, it can result in deafness.

• When the three little bones behind the eardrum fuse (a process called **otosclerosis**), they can no longer transmit the vibration of the eardrum produced by sounds entering the ear canal. This results in hearing loss and tinnitus. When otosclerosis is surgically corrected, hearing is restricted and tinnitus usually improves.

• **Repeated exposure to loud noise** sets you up for hearing loss and tinnitus later on. If you already have tinnitus, loud noise worsens it.

• **Hypothyroidism,** the underfunctioning of the thyroid gland, causes a host of symptoms such as dry skin, fluid retention, fatigue, sensitivity to cold, constipation, sluggishness—and tinnitus. These head noises are probably caused by swelling of the tissues in the inner ear. It's amazing how a little thyroid pill to replace the missing hormone can cure all these symptoms.

• **Infections** of the respiratory tract, especially those involving the ear drum—common colds and the flu, with and without fever—can cause tinnitus. It usually subsides when the infection is over.

• **If you're a tooth clencher or grinder,** you'll end up with a bad bite, worn-down teeth, problems with your temperomandibular joint (TMJ)—and tinnitus. Your dentist or oral surgeon can relieve the problem.

• **High cholesterol** and/or abnormal levels of other

blood fats are associated with tinnitus, presumably because they accelerate hardening of the arteries. Keeping your lipid profile as close to normal as possible, either by diet or drugs, may prevent tinnitus, but frankly, I've never seen it reverse this symptom.

How to Treat the Tinnitus of Aging

If all of the above possibilities have been corrected and your tinnitus is due to aging, here are some things to try:

A type of masking device is a good way to deal with troublesome tinnitus. These instruments make tinnitus more tolerable in at least 65 percent of cases. Most of them fit in your ear like a hearing aid and generate a more pleasant and acceptable noise than the tinnitus. You can make the sound from the device louder or softer as the situation demands, and you can even vary its pitch or tone. Make sure that the FDA has approved the unit you're planning to buy. A faulty one can affect your hearing over the long term.

William Shatner, in the depths of despair with his tinnitus, sought the help of a distinguished researcher in the field, Pawel Jastreboff, at the University of Maryland in Baltimore. Jastreboff has developed a masking device that produces "white noise"—a full spectrum of frequencies that sounds like the static between stations on your FM dial. Listening to this sound several hours a day for as long as a year and a half, and sometimes longer, desensitizes patients to the unwanted sound of their tinnitus. Shatner, like 80 percent of the patients treated this way, was helped so much by this treatment that he has become an enthusiastic spokesman for Dr. Jastreboff's clinic.

A hearing aid can also help tinnitus by amplifying environmental sounds that are usually more acceptable than the infernal tinnitus.

Alprazolam, better known as Xanax, widely used for the treatment of anxiety disorders, improves tinnitus in as many as 76 percent of cases. If the noise is getting you down, antidepressants, either the older tricyclics such as Elavil, or the newer selective serotonin uptake inhibitors (Prozac, Paxil, Zoloft) can make the symptoms more tolerable.

Although large doses of furosemide (Lasix), a potent diuretic (water pill), can cause tinnitus, this drug can also improve it in low dosages.

Biofeedback therapy helps some patients with troublesome tinnitus.

Chronic exposure to loud sounds (music, power tools, and other industrial noises) aggravates tinnitus. Avoid them when you can, and wear earmuffs or ear plugs when you can't.

Desperate patients sometimes ask me about surgical procedures that cut the nerve fibers associated with hearing. I have never found any of them to work and do not recommend them.

Homeopathy, acupuncture, chiropractic, and other non-mainstream techniques are of no proven benefit in treating tinnitus—except perhaps for *Ginkgo biloba*.

Made from the leaves of the ginkgo tree, this herb is the most widely prescribed "natural" product in Germany, where doctors write some 5 million prescriptions for it every year. Several reports in the European medical literature conclude that ginkgo is effective against tinnitus because it increases blood flow to the head. There has been very little research done in this country on ginkgo, despite the high degree of consumer interest in it. Given the few alternatives available, I have no hesitation about recommending it for anyone with tinnitus. However, ask your doctor for clearance before you start it. Ginkgo has an antiplatelet action similar to aspirin's, so it may make your blood too "thin" if you're taking aspirin in large doses or are on anticoagulants.

What to Remember about Tinnitus

1. Tinnitus (noise that originates in the head) affects at least 40 million people of all ages in this country.
2. Tinnitus should always be thoroughly investigated because it can be due to several remediable causes such as injuries to and infections of the ear, drugs, allergies, nicotine, caffeine, and alcohol. When these are corrected or removed, tinnitus usually disappears.
3. Tinnitus that accompanies the aging process is probably due to damage to the hair cells in the inner ear (also responsible for high-tone deafness, presbycusis).

4. Tinnitus due to aging is usually not curable, but
    there are ways to reduce its severity. The mainstays
    of therapy are various masking devices that substi-
    tute more pleasant sounds for the troublesome ones.
    Anti-anxiety agents and antidepressants can also
    help.

18

TOOTH LOSS
Gum Again?

When I was growing up, our family lived in a rather small apartment. There was only one bathroom, which my brother and I shared with my parents. On the shelf that held the soap, toothbrushes, and sponges, there was always a glass of water with my father's false teeth. I assumed them to be an inevitable consequence of aging, much like gray hair, and fully expected that, like my father, uncles, aunts, and, indeed, most "adults" I knew, I too would one day have them. (My mother, the insomniac [see Chapter 8] was the sole exception. She kept every single one of her teeth until she died at the age of ninety-four!) For me, dentures were a badge of maturity—the reward grown-ups reaped that freed them from the dentist's drill. I used to fantasize how wonderful it would be to have my own removable teeth that I could slip into my mouth before meals, remove after I no longer needed to chew, and then drop into a glass of water—free forever from toothaches, and the need to brush and floss after every meal.

Dental Decay and Tooth Loss

Fewer people have false teeth these days than when I was a child. You can realistically look forward to retaining most of your own teeth for as long as you live—unless, of course, you knock them out in an accident.

Remember when you were a child and had to go to the dentist every few months to have your cavities filled? My children suffered through fewer visits than I did, and my lucky grandchildren don't even know what a dentist's drill is! These days over half the kids ages five to seventeen have no tooth decay in their permanent teeth. Such dental health in childhood goes a long way toward assuring strong teeth in old age.

Fluoride, the magic ingredient responsible for conquering childhood cavities, has been added to our water supply and our toothpaste for the past forty years. Regardless of how the fluoride gets to your teeth—directly from your toothpaste, from fluoride gel applied directly to your teeth, or from the bloodstream after you've swallowed it—it strengthens tooth enamel, leaving it less vulnerable to attack by bacteria. Fluoride is as important for adults as it is for kids because decay does not respect age.

Dental decay at any age is caused by "bad" bacteria in the mouth that cling to the enamel of the teeth. When these bugs make contact with the sugar in our food, they form an acid that penetrates the enamel and makes it porous. When left untreated, this decay spreads through the softer material beneath the enamel and infects the interior of the tooth, the pulp, that contains nerves and blood vessels. When that happens, you need root-canal treatment to remove the infection to save the tooth.

Plaque, Tartar, and Gum Disease

Although dental decay in childhood is not as common as it used to be, tartar and plaque still are. Plaque is the sticky, colorless film of bacteria and other debris in the mouth that clings to the teeth. For the first twenty-four hours after it forms, you can get rid of it by brushing. If you wait any longer, the plaque hardens to form tartar or calculus, a rough, porous deposit that only your dentist or hygienist can remove by scraping. The bacteria in plaque and tartar attack the calcium and phosphorus in the enamel of the teeth and erode it. Plaque and tartar can also cause disease of the gums and the jawbone that holds the teeth. The gum disorder called chronic periodontitis starts as gingivitis, irritation and infection of the gums (the gingiva). Sixty percent of teenagers have gingivitis, as do half the adults in this country over the age of forty-five, and an even higher percentage of older persons.

Unless your dentist treats your gingivitis promptly, it ultimately leads to periodontal disease, in which the gums separate from the teeth, exposing their roots and forming pockets of infection where bacteria can multiply. As the infection spreads, it erodes the bone of the jaw, the teeth become loose and ultimately fall out. More than 60 percent of all forty-six-to-fifty-four-year-olds have some periodontal disease, as do 80 percent of those over age sixty-five.

Causes of Gum Disease

• **The bacterial kingpin** that causes periodontal disease is an organism called *P. gingiva*, of which there are different strains with varying degrees of aggressiveness. *P. gingiva* often infects several members of a household; 75 percent of spouses harbor identical strains in their mouths. These bacteria are transmitted by frequent kissing and sharing of eating utensils. However, whether you end up infected after such contact depends not only on the nature and extent of exposure, the aggressiveness of the particular strain, and the level of your resistance, but, most important, whether or not you have the pockets in your gums in which the organism can settle and multiply.

P. gingiva and other mouth pathogens in dental plaque may result in another totally unrelated complication. When you brush your teeth, some of these oral bacteria enter the bloodstream, where they cause the platelets to clump together. When this clumping affects the coronary arteries, it can, at least theoretically, result in clot formation! It all sounds a bit far-fetched to me, but it has been suggested that this may be the reason why heart attacks are so common in the early morning. But before you stop brushing your teeth in order to save your heart, let's wait for more research.

Periodontal disease may require gum surgery. However, a new antibiotic delivery system makes it possible to tuck the antibiotic directly into the diseased gum and leave it there to eradicate the infection. The ideal solution, one that is currently being investigated, would be a vaccine against the bacteria that cause gingivitis and periodontitis in the first place.

Receding gums and their subsequent infection are not the only causes of gingivitis. Medications can also inflame your gums. The most troublesome ones are the calcium channel blockers (nifedipine, diltiazem, verapamil) and their numerous derivatives, which are used in the treatment of high blood pressure and certain cardiac disorders, cyclosporin (the anti-rejection drug), dilantin (for the treatment of epilepsy), steroids, anticancer drugs, and some oral contraceptives.

• **Poorly fitting bridges,** or badly aligned teeth, promote plaque formation. So be sure to keep your dental appliances scrupulously clean.

If you clench or grind your teeth at night (a habit of which you are probably not aware), the excessive biting force will not only wear them down, but it will also speed up the loss of supporting bone. If your jaws are sore in the morning when you awaken or your spouse tells you you're grinding all night, let your dentist know. Wearing a mouth guard at night solves the problem.

• **Diabetes** in particular, as well as any other chronic disease such as AIDS, can reduce your resistance and lead to periodontal infection.

Signs of Gum Trouble

The first sign of gum trouble is bleeding after brushing. Other manifestations are redness, swelling, and tenderness of the gums, often accompanied by bad breath. Here are some other danger signals: When you run your finger from the gum to the biting edge of the tooth, it should feel smooth all the way. A bump or ridge across the width of the tooth suggests that your gums have receded and that you're in danger of losing the tooth. Now, open your mouth and look in the mirror (you don't have to say "Aah"). Yellow discoloration at the base of a tooth suggests that its root is exposed because of receding gums. (If you're a smoker, all your teeth are probably yellow. The gums may or may not be receding yet, but if you continue to smoke, chances are they will.) If you have any old crowns in your mouth and the teeth adjacent to them are darker, have your gums checked. However, discoloration of older teeth doesn't necessarily mean they're going to fall out. And don't waste your money on over-the-counter tooth whiteners. I don't think they work. Ask your dentist to bleach any discoloration that's cosmetically unacceptable to you.

How to Prevent Tooth Loss

Here's how to keep tartar and plaque under control:

• **Brush your teeth** with a soft- or medium-bristle brush at least twice a day, and preferably after every meal. (A soft brush is more effective than a hard one because it massages the gums as you brush, and it also gets into the crevices more effectively.) Use toothpaste that contains fluoride. Brush vertically in short strokes, four or five times, holding the toothbrush at a forty-five-degree angle against your gums. Brush all parts of your teeth—outer, inner, and chewing surfaces. When cleaning the inside surface of the front teeth, move the tip of the brush up and down gently. While you're at it, brush your tongue and gums, too, to get rid of odor-causing bacteria. The point of brushing is to clean your teeth, not to wipe them, so brush for at least three full minutes.

• **Brushing the teeth at bedtime** is an American ritual. While that's better than not brushing at all, it's not as effective as doing so right after you eat. The point of brushing is to get rid of the sugar that leads to plaque and tartar formation. If you eat dinner then wait for several hours before cleaning your teeth, sugar remains in contact with your teeth all that time. I'm not suggesting that you should excuse yourself when eating out in order to hunt for a washroom where you can brush your teeth. But when you're dining at home, brush right after dessert. Brush after breakfast, too. Most people brush when they awaken, to freshen the taste in their mouths. They then have breakfast and leave for work—without brushing. The right way is to rinse your mouth when you awaken, then brush after breakfast. Between meals, avoid snacks and drinks that contain sugar and cooked starches. They just sit there until the next scheduled brushing. Electric toothbrushes such as Interplak, Braun Oral-B, and Water-Pik may be more effective than ordinary toothbrushes, and they have the seal of approval of the American Dental Association—but you still need to brush for the same three minutes.

• **Flossing:** Even if you brush meticulously for a full three minutes, you'll still remove only 80 percent of the fresh plaque off your teeth. That's why flossing is so necessary. My dentist has two signs in his office that read ONLY FLOSS THOSE TEETH YOU WANT TO KEEP and IGNORE YOUR TEETH AND THEY'LL GO AWAY. Good advice. Here's the right way to floss: Use about eighteen inches of floss, either waxed or unwaxed. Wind most of it around the middle finger of one hand and the rest around the same finger of the other hand. Holding the floss tight between your thumb and forefinger, move it between your teeth, up around the gum, then down along the tooth. From time to time, unwind some clean floss off one finger and take up the used floss with the other.

It's all very well for me to advise you to brush vigorously and floss regularly, but that's easier said than done if you have severe arthritis of the hands, Parkinson's disease, multiple sclerosis, or any neurological disorder that impairs your movement. If you have such a problem, an electric or sonic toothbrush can help.

• **Your dentist (or hygienist) or periodontist should clean your teeth,** deep-scale the plaques and tartar, and plane the root surfaces of the teeth below the gum line at least twice a year. If you're a plaque maker, however, you may need it done more often than that. My periodontist has me come back every three months, but then he's putting three children through college.

• **Ask your dentist about mouth rinses** that contain the antibacterial agent chlorhexidine (Peridex—by prescription only) or preparations with eucalyptol, menthol, methyl salicylate, and thymol. Chlorhexidine reduces plaque by 55 percent and gingivitis by 45 percent, but it discolors the teeth in some people, especially when they use a full-strength version that's not diluted. I prefer Listerine antiseptic; it's somewhat less effective—it cuts plaque by 28 percent and gingivitis by 30 percent—but it doesn't require a prescription and won't stain your teeth.

• **Look for a toothpaste** like Total that, in addition to the usual fluoride, contains triclosan. This is an antibacterial agent that adheres to the teeth after brushing, reduces the accumulation of tartar and plaque, and helps prevent infection of the gums. My dentist is not convinced that toothpaste containing baking soda or peroxide has any special advantage, but my wife's dentist swears by it!

• **Saliva** rinses away food particles and neutralizes harmful acids. However, as we get older, our mouths are not as juicy, so that the gums become more vulnerable to infection. Several medications can cause oral dryness, notably diuretics (water pills), a variety of antihistamines, blood pressure–lowering agents, decongestants, and tranquilizers. Certain disorders such as Sjogren's can also dehydrate the mouth. Whatever the cause, chewing gum (preferably the sugarless variety), although it may not be the most elegant thing to do, does increase the production of saliva. And here's a tip for dealing with dry mouth I'll bet you never heard of: Cheese, especially cheddar, neutralizes the acid produced by bacteria and increases the flow of saliva. After-dinner mints or candy that you see in those large bowls near the front door of the restaurants when you're leaving may freshen your breath, but they coat your teeth with sugar that sits there until you get home. If you have a choice, take the toothpicks they offer and stay away from the mints.

• **Tobacco** doubles the risk of your becoming edentulous by hindering your immune response and by decreasing blood flow to the gums. If you smoke one pack a day, expect to lose two teeth every ten years.

• **Estrogen replacement therapy (ERT)** after menopause not only helps prevent osteoporosis, it also prevents tooth loss by minimizing the leak of calcium from the jawbone. This significantly reduces your chances of ending up toothless. In a study of 4,000 retirement-aged women, those who had taken estrogen for fifteen years were at half the risk of becoming edentulous as compared to those who used no supplements at all.

When Prevention Fails

• **Sealants:** Since fluoride protects the flat areas of the teeth, most decay now occurs in the pits and fissures that form on their chewing surfaces. These areas can now be protected by resinous sealants that harden when applied to the teeth by a dentist. These materials are particularly effective for cavity control in children because so many adults already have metal fillings to which the resins do not adhere nearly as well. However, as you will see below, sealants have other uses in older persons.

As you get older, your teeth may become discolored or damaged, or lose some height; their edges may be sharper or flatter, especially if your "bite" (how your teeth line up when you chew) is off or if you grind them at night. Or you may have lost some teeth, so that you now resemble a jack-o'-lantern when you smile. In the "old days," your only option to improve your appearance was to remove the offending teeth. If a few stragglers were left behind, it was easier to have them pulled and replaced with a complete set of dentures. That's still an option, but certainly not the only one, thanks to the development of bonding and dental implants. This is good news for the four out of every ten Americans over age sixty-five who have lost all their teeth, and the millions of adults who wear dentures because they're missing several of them.

• **Bonding,** a technique using composite resins (see above) corrects stains and restores cracked, discolored, or chipped teeth. It's called "bonding" because the materials applied to the teeth bond with the enamel, strengthening them so they tolerate the pressures created by chewing and biting. This technique usually involves molding a soft resin or porcelain veneer to the front of the tooth (it's much like putting on false fingernails). Once it's hardened, the coating can either be left as a simple cover or the dentist can grind it to a specific shape, restoring or improving the original appearance of the tooth. The older techniques of capping and crowning damaged teeth required grinding them down and then securing them to a post. Bonding is preferable because it leaves teeth in their natural state.

Bonding can also secure bridgework. Traditionally, in order to place a false tooth between two natural teeth, the dentist filed down your natural teeth, then covered them with a device, the middle of which carries the replacement tooth. With bonding, if the teeth on either side of the false one are strong enough, the replacement tooth can be attached to them without grinding.

Bonding has other advantages: It costs half as much as older bridges and crowns, it's much quicker (four or five teeth can be bonded in the time it takes to prepare and apply one crown), and it's often reversible if you don't care for the result. Until recently, dentists bonded only the front teeth. Newer materials are now available that make bonding more durable, easier to match up with the color and shape of the other teeth, less prone to discoloration, and that can be used to bond the back teeth, too. The molars take the biggest beating biting, so if you have any of your front teeth bonded, do not bite into an apple or carrot, or anything hard, and avoid caramels. You may note some staining of the bonded front teeth if you're a tea or coffee drinker. That was particularly embarrassing for me when patients asked whether the slightly yellow tinge on my front teeth was from cigarette smoking. Imagine me smoking!

The benefits of bonding far outweigh its disadvantages. If you have a choice, bonding is the way to go.

• **Hundreds of thousands of Americans have dental implants,** one of the major breakthroughs in dentistry. These implants are usually the best way to replace missing teeth, small bridges, or removable partial dentures. Metal screws are placed into the jawbone, where they serve as an anchor for artificial teeth. You've got to have good strong bone into which to put the screw (or "post," as it is called). The best results are obtained from implants in the front part of the lower jaw, although chances of the procedure being successful are high (85 to 90 percent) virtually anywhere in the mouth. The procedure is done under local anesthesia so it doesn't hurt, although when the Novocaine wears off in a few hours, your mouth may ache for a while. Implants are usually made of titanium.

Implants are expensive. A complete set of artificial teeth can easily set you back more than $10,000. And don't kid yourself: As good as they are, they're not quite like your own teeth. Depending on the number of teeth to be replaced, a commitment to implants may require many visits over a period of several months, and lots of surgery. There will be days when you won't be able to eat solid food, when your gums will hurt, and when you'll be wearing temporary devices. Once the job is done, you'll need to follow special oral hygiene instructions for the rest of your life. You may not even be a suitable candidate for implant surgery if you have diabetes, high blood pressure, any chronic illness, if you're taking blood thinners (anticoagulants), if you have valvular heart disease and are vulnerable to infection of the heart valves (endocarditis), or if you're a heavy smoker or drinker, or grind your teeth especially vigorously at night. All these conditions can prevent a good long-term result. Even otherwise healthy persons can suffer complications from implant procedures: infection at the site of the surgery, even perforation of the bone, and rejection of the implant. These problems are more likely to occur if your dentist is not as skilled as he or she might be. However, despite all these real and potential drawbacks, implants are the best way to deal with tooth loss.

The major advantage of implants over removable dentures and bridges is that implants are fixed and stable, while the others are apt to wobble in your mouth. (Some have even fallen into my lap while I was examining an edentulous patient's throat.) Dentures present the greatest problem when you eat, speak, or, worst of all, yawn. Some of the newer dental adhesives do help matters somewhat, but not as much as the late Mary Martin and the other TV advertisers would have you believe. Another drawback to dentures is the food that lodges in, around, and under the appliance (the reason my father kept his in a glass of water when he wasn't using them).

It's crucial that your dental implant be done right. That requires skill, training, and experience. Check the qualifications of the person you've chosen to do the job. Although some general dentists or prosthodontists (the people who make crowns and dentures) can place implants, I refer my own patients to specialist oral surgeons or periodontists.

There are basically two types of implants: on-the-bone

(now done only rarely) and in-the-bone. When applying an on-the-bone implant, the dentist cuts the gums, fits a frame onto the bone, and then sews the gum back. Posts on the frame protrude through the gum, and the teeth or bridge are attached to them. The in-the-bone implant doesn't sit on the bone but is implanted into it. The implant has a screw hole in its center into which screws are placed to anchor one or more artificial teeth, or entire rows of replacements.

While implants are the best way to deal with tooth loss, they're not always easy to do. Remember, there's nothing as good as your own teeth. Before accepting any artificial ones, make sure you've done everything possible to save your own.

What to Remember about Tooth Loss

1. Tooth loss and the prospect of dentures are no longer inevitable.
2. Fluoridation has virtually eliminated childhood tooth decay; the most important remaining cause of tooth loss as you age is gum disease.
3. Gum disease can be prevented by proper brushing and flossing of the teeth, as well as regular visits to the dentist for the removal of tartar and plaque.
4. Gum infections are caused by bacteria in plaques that may be transmitted through kissing.
5. Special mouth rinses and toothpastes can reduce plaque formation and gum disease.

6. Electric toothbrushes are more effective than the standard variety.
7. A decrease in saliva associated with age, and also caused by certain medications, predisposes to gum infection and tooth loss.
8. Estrogen replacement therapy in post-menopausal women reduces the risk of tooth loss by half.
9. New bonding techniques can repair damaged and discolored teeth, often eliminating the need for crowns, bridges, and dentures.
10. Dental implants can free you from the inconvenience of removable dentures. Although these procedures are superior to the removable devices, they are costly, time-consuming, and carry with them the risk of infection or rejection. They may not be suitable for persons with chronic illnesses.

19

LOSS OF VISION — MACULAR DEGENERATION, CATARACTS, AND GLAUCOMA

Loss of Vision

As we get older, most of us read with outstretched arms, holding our books and newspapers farther and farther away from our eyes. Unfortunately, nature did not make our arms long enough (that evolutionary design was wasted on orangutans, who don't even read). We finally capitulate and get eyeglasses. The prospect of wearing spectacles doesn't worry or depress most people, since glasses are no longer a stigma of old age; every child prodigy seems to wear them. And they don't make you look old, either—they can be as chic and sexy as you like. There's a style to suit every personality: designer frames if you're fashionable, a monocle if you're pompous (or Prussian), and lunettes if you're social. If you don't happen to care for spectacles, you can have contact lenses; they're inexpensive, safe, and easy to insert and remove. Not only do they correct your vision without advertising your impairment, they can even make your eyes the beautiful shade of blue (or any other color) you've always wanted. (Alas, hearing aids do not have the same acceptance and are still identified with old age. That's why so many of the hard of hearing keep trading theirs "up" for smaller and smaller, virtually invisible devices. Take a look at my picture on the jacket of this book. Can you see mine?)

The focus of this chapter is the prevention and treatment of macular degeneration, cataracts, and glaucoma—the three major, serious, age-related eye disorders that cause most of the blindness or near-blindness among the elderly in our society. As is true for many "complications" of aging, you can almost always prevent them or at least reduce your chances of developing them. And even if you are stricken, there are ways to treat them, to hold them in check, and sometimes even to cure them.

How We See

Although macular degeneration, cataracts, and glaucoma are totally different entities, they do have some risk factors in common. For you to prevent or manage them, you need to understand how and why they develop. So here's a short course on the mechanism of eyesight.

The rays of light that carry an image pass through the

cornea, the clear, transparent, outermost curved tissue of the eyeball that covers the colored portion of the eye, and then through the normally clear *lens* behind it. A healthy lens is elastic and biconvex, but can change its shape to accommodate different visual needs—looking at an object either close up or at a distance. The cornea and lens together focus the light (or image) onto the *retina,* a thin layer of light-sensitive tissue in the back of the eye. The retina contains millions of cells that convert the image into electrical impulses picked up by myriad nerve fibers that converge to form the *optic nerve.* The optic nerve delivers the final visual message to the brain, which interprets it for you. The *macula,* a tiny area several millimeters in diameter, is located in the middle of the retina and contains photoreceptors and nerve cells that are responsible for central vision and color perception.

Things can go wrong anywhere along the line. The cornea can become damaged, scarred, or opaque and block the passage of light through it; the lens too, instead of being crystal clear, can also become cloudy and dense and similarly interfere with the passage of light to the retina; the macula, which you need in order to read, drive, sew, and do all the things that require central vision, can degenerate; the rest of the retina can be damaged by blood vessels that have burst in the interior of the eye or that grow exuberantly within it; the optic nerve can become diseased and stop transmitting its messages to the brain; and finally, the brain itself can be injured by a stroke, a tumor, or another disease so that it loses its ability to receive and interpret information from the eye.

What Is Legal Blindness?

Let's define blindness before we discuss its major causes. You can't always tell how well someone sees just by looking at the person, even if he or she carries a white cane and has a Seeing Eye dog. In Venice last year, I saw a "blind" beggar, shabbily dressed, "feeling out" the sidewalk ahead of him with a white cane. A little girl was guiding him. This pathetic sight made me very sad, and I gave him a few lire to ease his plight. Later that afternoon, I saw him again in a different part of the city. He was wearing an expensive suit, walking briskly without a cane or a guide and accompanied by a well-dressed young woman. My original diagnosis was obviously wrong. This "beggar" was not blind. He was a "businessman," a professional con artist, earning a living from the compassion of strangers.

The legal definition of blindness in most states is "corrected vision no better than 20/200 in both eyes." That means you can see at no farther than 20 feet what a normal person can identify from a distance of 200 feet. (Corrected vision must be at least 20/40 in order to qualify for a driver's license.) You're also blind if you have a visual field of only 20 degrees. If you were to stand at the center of a large clock and look straight ahead at twelve o'clock, you couldn't see beyond the eleven o'clock or one o'clock markers on either side. However, for practical purposes, you're considered to be blind if you can't count the fingers held up by someone ten feet away in daylight.

The Magnitude of the Problem

Given these definitions, there are about 500,000 blind people in this country, and some 50,000 newcomers join their ranks every year. But that's only the tip of the iceberg because there are at least 10 million Americans who, though not legally blind, have seriously impaired eyesight. Almost 2 million can't make out the print in the newspaper even with glasses and other vision aids. Most of these sight problems are due to the three disorders described below:

Macular Degeneration: Looking Askew

Macular degeneration is the leading cause of significant permanent vision loss in this country. Some 3 million people can't see normally due to this disorder, and this figure is expected to triple by the year 2020 as the population ages. Macular degeneration affects an additional 165,000 persons every year, of whom 16,000 become legally blind. Virtually all of them are older than fifty-five; Caucasians are more frequently stricken than Blacks, and persons with light-colored eyes are especially vulnerable.

In someone with macular degeneration, tissues in the macula (the tiny area in the middle of the retina responsible for central and color vision), degenerate or break down. As a result, central vision (what you see when you look straight ahead) becomes distorted and blurred. You are also unable to differentiate one color from another. However, since the rest of the retina is not usually affected, you can still see out of the sides of your eyes. I remember wondering why my father always sat *beside* the TV and not in front of it. Now I know. Although someone with macular degeneration may not be able to read, drive, see a movie, or do close-up work, he or she is not necessarily legally blind.

TWO VERY DIFFERENT TYPES OF MACULAR DEGENERATION

There are two kinds of macular degeneration, each with its own outlook and treatment. In the *dry* form, which accounts for 90 percent of cases, the macular tissue breaks down gradually over the years, and the process speeds up or slows down unpredictably. Vision becomes blurred and is not helped much by new glasses. However, magnifying glasses and other visual aids do make a difference. This dry form rarely leads to legal blindness.

By contrast, the *wet* form of macular degeneration, which comprises only 10 percent of cases, causes 85 percent of the blindness due to this disorder. It's called "wet" because tiny blood vessels behind the macula begin to leak; the blood spreads into the surrounding areas and eventually forms scar tissue, which interferes with vision. New blood vessels form within this scar tissue in an attempt to help nourish it (a serious miscalculation by nature), reducing vision even more. The leaking blood and the scar tissue with its new, abnormal blood vessels all damage the macula. Sight is blurred and distorted; telephone poles seem to wave in the breeze, and when you look straight ahead you see only an empty space because the scar tissue has completely obstructed your central vision. Remember that side—peripheral—vision is not affected. Vision is worse if both eyes are affected, but you may see perfectly well if there is wet macular degeneration in only one eye, because the other healthy one compensates very well. However, both eyes usually become diseased in time.

Dry macular degeneration is easily diagnosed with the instruments used by ophthalmologists in their offices; the wet form usually requires more sophisticated procedures such as fluorescein angiography, in which dye is injected into the eye in order to highlight the blood vessels that are doing all the leaking and growing.

WHAT CAUSES MACULAR DEGENERATION?

You can reduce your risk of developing macular degeneration if you understand how and why it comes about. Normal use of your eyes won't cause it; neither will long hours of reading or looking up at the stars. And there's no correlation with high blood sugar or cholesterol levels, either. The important risk factors are:

• **Genetics:** Scientists believe they may have found the gene responsible for dry macular degeneration, and expect that in the foreseeable future they will be able to treat what is now an incurable disease. You can't choose your genes, but if other members of your family have macular degeneration, you're vulnerable and should concentrate all the harder to eliminate the factors that are under your control.

• **Pollution is important.** That's why the incidence of macular degeneration is much lower in the pristine environment of southern Italy than in central London. Although other factors may play a role in these two areas, air quality is obviously a key determinant. Macular degeneration is the most common cause of blindness in Japan because of the proliferation of industrial wastes and fumes. This eye disease was virtually unknown there only twenty years ago.

• **Diet:** A lifetime of eating lots of fat and too few fruits and vegetables makes you a good candidate for macular degeneration. Some eye specialists also believe that the widespread use of plastics has contaminated our food with polyphenols, chemicals that promote the breakdown of body tissues such as the macula.

• **Cigarette smoking** is a major villain. Tobacco reduces blood flow to the eyes. In the ongoing Nurses' Health Study that's now been conducted for many years at Harvard Medical School, women who smoked at least twenty-five cigarettes per day had 2.4 times the incidence of macular degeneration of the abstainers.

• **Sun:** A lifetime of excessive, unprotected exposure to bright sunlight is a major cause of macular degeneration. Light is believed to activate oxygen metabolism in the eye, resulting in the overproduction of free radicals that damage the macular tissues (in the same way they hurt other organs throughout the body).

• **Other aggravators:** While the data are conflicting, high blood pressure and cardiovascular disease do not seem to cause macular degeneration, but they may make it more difficult to control.

HOW TO PREVENT MACULAR DEGENERATION

You must avoid or control the factors believed to cause macular degeneration in order to reduce the chances of developing it.

• **Pollution** is everyone's responsibility—government, industry, and individuals.

• **Protect your eyes against sunlight** starting early in life. The sun gives off several kinds of rays: visible light, which we need in order to see; infrared rays, which are invisible and create heat; and ultraviolet rays. The latter are the most harmful, and consist of three main varieties, A, B, and blue light. Chronic exposure to ultraviolet rays, especially the B spectrum, not only promotes macular degeneration, but, as you will see later, it also predisposes to cataracts and cancer of the skin around the eyes. (Short-term intense exposure causes photokeratitis, a painful ocular irritation.) Ultraviolet radiation is now more deadly than ever because the protective ozone layer that shields us from it is gradually melting away.

We receive 80 percent of our total lifetime exposure to the harmful rays of the sun during the first eighteen years of life. When you're young, the lens of the eye is crystal clear and doesn't filter any of the ultraviolet rays, especially the dangerous "blue light" that damages the retina. So it's especially important to protect your children from them. Make sure that you and your kids wear sunglasses in bright light, especially at the beach, or in any environment such as snowy mountain slopes where there is lots of glare.

You can't judge the effectiveness of sunglasses by their color or their price. Designer glasses may be chic and expensive, but they don't necessarily protect you. When buying sunglasses, make sure the label states that they block 99 to 100 percent of ultraviolet A and B (UV-A, UV-B). If you're getting prescription sunglasses, be sure to specify to the optometrist exactly what you want. The glasses should wrap around and fit closely; otherwise the rays get in from the side.

• **The right diet** can help prevent macular degeneration and/or slow its progress. Foods rich in zinc as well as antioxidant vitamins such as A, C, and E probably help protect against the dry form. Try to get these vitamins and other antioxidants from natural sources, if possible. You'll find them in dark green vegetables such as spinach, broccoli (I read recently that the distaste for broccoli that some people, and presidents, have may be genetically determined), kale, brussels sprouts, leaf lettuce, celery, and collard greens. Five to nine servings a day can lower your risk of developing macular degeneration. That may sound like a lot, but remember that one cup of berries or a spinach salad each equals two servings. These foods are protective because two of their ingredients, lutein and zeaxanthin, are antioxidants that are also normally present in high concentrations in the retina. They act as free-radical scavengers, cleansing the retinal and macular areas of waste products that cause tissue breakdown. (Beta-carotene supplements have no lutein or zeaxanthin.) Researchers at Harvard found that 6 milligrams of lutein daily decreased the incidence of macular degeneration.

The National Eye Institute is currently conducting long-term studies of the role of antioxidants in the development of macular degeneration, but their results will not be available for several years. Don't wait. Load up on these foods right now.

• On a more practical and pleasant note, there is some evidence that two to twelve glasses of wine *per year* can reduce the incidence of macular degeneration by as much as almost 50 percent. (As an oenophile, I consider this to be a ridiculously small amount.) Wine is thought to provide this protection by interfering with the action of platelets that increase the stickiness of the blood so that it clots less easily, and also by its antioxidant effects.

• I was impressed by a study reported in 1996 in the *Journal of the American Optometric Association* in which patients with early macular degeneration who were given zinc supplements had much slower progression of their disease than did those who received placebos. Zinc is normally present in high concentrations in the retina and the tissues surrounding the macula, and activates the enzymes that facilitate certain biochemical processes in most tissues of the body, including the eye. Older persons are zinc-deprived, either because they don't absorb it as well from their aging intestinal tract or because they don't eat enough of the foods that contain it, such as beef and fish. Many eye doctors prescribe zinc supplements to patients with macular degeneration. Take 25 or 50 milligrams of a zinc supplement a day.

TREATING MACULAR DEGENERATION

The dry form of macular degeneration progresses insidiously over the years, and there is very little you can do about it other than the dietary measures described above. However, lasers can often help the wet form. Fluorescein dye is injected into the eye to identify the leaking blood vessels, after which they can be sealed with a laser beam. New blood vessels that have formed in scar tissue can be "burned" with the beam. These procedures do not cure macular degeneration because nothing can remove the scar tissue, revitalize the destroyed macula, or restore vision, but they often slow down the course of the disease. The sooner treatment is begun, the better the results.

WHAT TO REMEMBER ABOUT
MACULAR DEGENERATION

1. Macular degeneration is the most important cause of serious vision loss in persons older than sixty years. Since it only affects central and color vision, you can still see from the sides of your eyes.

2. There are two different types of macular degeneration—the dry and the wet. Their management and outlook differ; the former is much more common but less serious.

3. Frequent and prolonged exposure to the harmful rays of the sun is a risk factor for macular degeneration. It's important for you and your children always to wear sunglasses in bright sunlight.

4. People who live in a polluted environment or who smoke cigarettes are more prone to macular degeneration.

5. There is growing evidence that antioxidant vitamins such as A, C, and E, as well as leafy green vegetables and zinc supplements, can prevent or slow down the progression of dry macular degeneration.

6. Laser therapy can retard the deterioration of the wet form, which often starts suddenly and gets rapidly worse; the dry form progresses slowly over the years and is best treated by diet.

Cataracts: Oh, Say, Can You See?

Cataracts are the third leading cause of legal blindness in the United States, and their surgical removal from over 2 million people every year (the only way to cure them) makes this the most commonly performed operation in America. It also takes the biggest bite—$3.2 billion annually—out of the nation's Medicare budget. Although the young can develop cataracts too, usually as a result of injury or a congenital disorder, in this chapter I will be describing only cataracts that are associated with aging.

Cataract refers to the clouding or opacification of the lens of the eye. The lens is a biconvex structure, rounded outward on both sides, like a compressed sphere. It lies behind the cornea and the colored part of the eye, the iris. The lens focuses the light image that enters the eye onto the retina. Because it's elastic, the lens can change its shape when necessary, making it possible for you to shift your gaze quickly from some distant object to the fine print of your newspaper—and still be in focus.

The lens is made up of just the right proportions of water and protein, and is crystal clear for the first years of life. It permits light to pass unhindered through it to the back of the eye. But when we reach the forties or fifties, the lens' protein begins to become milky and cloudy—the first stage of a cataract. By age seventy-five, it's opaque enough to interfere with normal vision. From then on it's usually just a matter of time before it has to be extracted.

You know your cataract is ready to come out when you feel like you're looking through a waterfall. (The word *cataract* means "waterfall.") Fortunately, although cataracts usually affect both eyes, they usually do so at different rates. You can therefore have one removed, assess the results of the surgery and have the other one done later at your convenience.

A little anatomy lesson here will help you understand how, when, and why cataracts are treated. There are three parts to the lens: a *capsule* that wraps around the *cortex,* whose center consists of a *nucleus.* It's like a peach, with its skin, fleshy part, and pit. Any one or all of these components of the lens can be affected. Cataracts due to simple aging usually affect the nucleus (nuclear cataract); diabetics tend to form cataracts in the cortex (cortical cataract) or the capsule (subcapsular cataract); persons with high myopia (shortsightedness), or who have taken steroid hormones for long periods of time, are most likely to develop subcapsular cataracts.

WHAT CAUSES THE AGING CATARACT, AND HOW CAN YOU PREVENT IT?

There's a common misperception that normal use of your eyes, voracious reading, and sitting too close and too long in front of the TV cause cataracts. That's eyewash! Nor are cataracts a natural and inevitable accompaniment of aging that you can do nothing to prevent.

Here are some causes of accelerated cataract formation; some are unavoidable, but several are under your control:

- **Smoking** triples the risk. Quit now.
- **Excessive alcohol** consumption makes you more vulnerable.
- **Overweight** increases the risk.
- **Diabetes,** with prolonged periods of elevated sugar, promotes cataract formation. Try to keep your blood sugar as close to normal as possible.
- **Chronically elevated blood pressure** is a risk factor for cataracts. No one knows why some hypertensives develop them and others don't. But high blood pressure is easy to treat; you should not be walking around with abnormal readings.
- **Abnormal blood-fat levels** (e.g., high cholesterol) predispose you to cataracts. The right diet, and, if necessary, one of the new, safe, and effective medications that help bring your cholesterol and LDL (the bad cholesterol) down to normal readings can reduce the risk of cataracts.
- **Many people require oral steroids** (drugs belonging to the cortisone family) to manage their asthma, cancer, arthritis, or to prevent rejection of their organ transplants. Long-term use of steroids definitely causes cataracts. However, abandoning them can lead to more serious consequences than cataracts. Inhaled steroids, used to control an acute asthmatic attack, make cataracts two to five times more likely. Here too, it's more important to treat the life-threatening symptoms than to worry about the potential risk of cataract formation.

• **Increased, unprotected exposure to solar ultra-violet radiation** (UV-B) is an important cause of cataracts. You can avoid excessive exposure by keeping out of the sun and wearing wide-brimmed hats and good sunglasses outdoors.

• **A diet poor in fruits and vegetables** sets you up for cataracts later in life. Antioxidants in the form of fruits and vegetables (seven to nine servings a day) are protective. Supplemental vitamin C may be beneficial. In one report, women who took 250 to 500 milligrams of vitamin C daily for ten years or more had a 77 percent lower incidence of cataracts than those who did not. In another study, taking supplemental vitamin C and E delayed the need for cataract surgery by as much as ten years. These antioxidants help prevent cataract formation by removing free radicals from the lens. When these waste products of oxidation accumulate, the lens undergoes biochemical changes that opacify it. Some ophthalmologists also recommend supplements of copper, selenium, beta-carotene, and the antioxidant L-glutathione (available in health-food stores), as well as one drop of zinc ascorbate in each eye twice a day. However, I'm not aware of any proof that any of these measures help.

• **Living at high altitude** is a risk factor for cataracts. The low oxygen content of the atmosphere is presumably responsible for accelerating cataract formation.

• **Chronic use of diuretics** (water pills) promotes cataract formation. However, the threat to you from the conditions for which diuretics are prescribed is usually greater than that posed by cataracts.

• **Chronic use of major tranquilizers** may enhance cataracts. But, once again, whether or not you take these or any medication should not be determined by the risk of their giving you cataracts.

SYMPTOMS OF A CATARACT

Suspect a cataract if your vision has become a little blurry, as if you're looking through a cloudy window. Cleaning your glasses carefully, which is what most people do, doesn't help (unless, of course, in addition to a cataract, you also have dirty spectacles). Cataracts also make the light seem harshly bright and glaring whether it's from the sun or from your reading lamp. There is often a halo when you look at a lightbulb. The headlights of every oncoming car appear to be on the "bright" setting. As your cataract gets worse, colors appear less brilliant, reading small print becomes more and more difficult, and pretty soon a magnifying glass becomes as important to you as your regular glasses. Finally, you end up seeing through a "waterfall."

TREATING AND REMOVING YOUR CATARACT

The only way to get rid of a cataract is to remove it surgically. No eye drops will make it disappear, and, once it's formed, neither will diet, special exercises, or other lifestyle changes. Changing glasses will work only for so long; they cannot penetrate a densely clouded lens. But don't have the operation to remove an early cataract. You can buy some time by changing your glasses. Stronger bifocals will also help, as will a magnifying glass for the fine print. Doctors used to advise waiting until the cataract "ripens." There's no such thing. The time should be "ripe" for you, not for your doctor or your cataract. You're ready for surgery when your vision is so poor that it affects the quality of your life—you don't see well enough to do your household chores, read books and the newspaper, make out the labels on your medication bottles, watch TV, go out with friends, do your job. If you've been stumbling and falling because you can't see where you're going or if you can no longer drive a car, then it's surely time. But when to have a cataract out is entirely up to you—and only you. If you choose to wait and you're comfortable doing so, nothing dire will happen to the cataract. It's never too late for surgery.

HOW SHOULD YOUR CATARACT BE REMOVED?

Cataract surgery is usually a same-day procedure. I remember when it used to take hours to do and patients were kept in the hospital for days or weeks, blindfolded until their eyes healed. The only inconvenience these days is missing breakfast the day of your surgery. You probably won't need general anesthesia, but you will be given a tranquilizer to help you relax. Most patients receive an injection into the eye, but in some cases anesthetic eye drops will do. Chances are you'll be sent home the same day with an eye shield (let someone else do the driving). You'll probably be able to read the very next day, but avoid contact sports for a few weeks.

Years ago, if you needed any operation, you asked around for the name of the best doctor and the rest was up to him. Times have changed. Find out from your ophthalmologist what procedure will be used.

There have been several major advances in the techniques of lens removal; you should know what they are, and how much experience your surgeon has had with them.

The purpose of a cataract operation is to get rid of the cloudy lens. That can be done in several ways. There is the "intracapsular" operation, the doctor makes an incision through the cornea and removes the cataract in one piece, along with the capsule that encloses it. This is an older method that should no longer be used. The incision to extract the cataract is much bigger than necessary by today's standards; it scars the cornea and leaves you with less than optimal vision. The best long-term results are obtained with the smallest surgical incision in the cornea because the smaller the slit, the less the astigmatism—visual distortion due to irregularities in the cornea.

The more recent "extracapsular capsular extraction" technique (ECCE) is much more preferable than the intracapsular procedure. The lens is removed but the capsule that envelops it is left intact. I prefer the ECCE technique with phacoemulsification ("phaco" for short), which has been in use since the 1980s. This requires the smallest cut, causes the least scarring, and leaves you with the best vision.

Phacoemulsification differs from the earlier ECCE method because, instead of extracting the cloudy lens, the doctor breaks it up into tiny pieces with high-frequency sound waves delivered by a small ultrasound probe. Only a small incision is then required to "vacuum" out the residue. Although some doctors will tell you that the size of the incision really makes no difference in the long run and that all ECCE methods are equally good (almost a half million of the older ones are still being done every year), the evidence suggests otherwise. When my cataract "ripens" and I can no longer see this keyboard, I will have it removed by phacoemulsification.

After your lens has been extracted, you need a new, artificial one, most of which are made of acrylic or silicone. Because they're flexible, they can be folded like a taco (I suggest that the whole procedure be called the phaco-taco operation) and easily inserted through a slit only three millimeters long. These foldable lenses take less time to heal than the older, rigid implants. The FDA has recently approved a new multifocus, foldable lens that has been used in Europe with great success. It allows you to see close up and read without glasses. Before your cataract surgery, ask your doctor to get one for you.

In those rare cases where the lens cannot be replaced because the patient is too debilitated or for other technical reasons, then either contact lenses or thick cataract glasses are used.

AFTER YOUR CATARACT HAS BEEN REMOVED

How well you will see after your cataract has been removed depends on the kind of operation you had and the type of lens that was implanted. Also, if you have some other underlying eye problem such as macular degeneration or glaucoma, or if there are hemorrhages in your eyes from poorly controlled diabetes or high blood pressure, no lens will restore perfect vision.

Will you still need glasses after your cataract surgery? Some people don't, but most do require reading glasses, or bifocals for distant vision.

After your lens has been removed the body can't grow another one, so don't worry about cataracts reforming. But half the patients undergoing ECCE or phacoemulsification need another procedure within two years because the lens capsule that is left behind can become cloudy. You'll know that's what's happened if you enjoyed excellent vision after the surgery but then the familiar cloudiness returned. This complication is treated by a YAG capsulotomy, in which the doctor makes a tiny opening in the back of the cloudy capsule with a laser beam. This permits light to pass through to the retina. The YAG capsulotomy takes only a few minutes and is an outpatient procedure.

WHAT TO REMEMBER ABOUT CATARACTS

1. Cataracts are the third leading cause of legal blindness in the United States. They are due to clouding of the normally transparent lens of the eye so that enough light does not reach the retina.
2. The major known contributing causes of cataracts are smoking, too much alcohol, chronic exposure to the ultraviolet rays of the sun, a diet lacking in vitamins C and E and fruits and vegetables, and long-term use of certain medications, especially steroid hormones.
3. The only way to treat cataracts is to remove the opaque lens and replace it with a synthetic one. This is no longer a big deal. You're in and out of the hospital the same day, and the operative risk is slight.
4. It is important to know what surgical method your doctor plans to use because the more modern techniques yield the best results. Although vision is almost always restored, chances are you'll probably need reading and/or distance glasses.
5. The timing of the operation is entirely up to you. There's no reason to rush into surgery as long as your visual problems are not interfering with the quality of your life.

Glaucoma: What's Your Angle?

Some 3 million people age forty and older (that's one in every thirty) have glaucoma—and half of them don't know it! It is the second leading cause of blindness in this country, accounting for 12 percent of all cases of blindness and affecting some 150,000 people, while impairing the eyesight of an additional 1.6 million Americans.

I recently ran into an old high-school friend whom I hadn't seen for a long time. After we caught up with the events of the past thirty-five years, he confided to me that he was very depressed. "My doctor gave me some bad news the other day. He found high pressure in my eyes during a routine eye exam. I was really surprised because my vision is perfect and I feel great. Anyway, it seems that I have high eye pressure, and I'll probably end up blind."

Like so many people, my friend simply assumed that because his intraocular pressure was high, he would inevitably develop glaucoma and lose his eyesight. *Elevated ocular pressure results in glaucoma only if it's been left untreated for any length of time.* Then and only then can it cause serious impairment of vision. It does so in only 30 percent of cases by damaging the optic nerve, which carries visual images to the brain. Nevertheless, we treat everyone with high eye pressure because there's no way of knowing who will become blind and who will not.

My friend was lucky. His increased ocular pressure was detected in time, treatment with medication had already been started, and he would, in fact, probably not develop glaucoma or ever go blind.

THE CAUSES AND SIGNS OF ELEVATED OCULAR PRESSURE

The interior of the eye is bathed in a clear, nourishing liquid that's constantly being produced by tissues around the lens. Aqueous humor (there's nothing funny about it) keeps the interior of the eye from drying out. Don't confuse it with tears, which are made *outside* of the eye and whose job it is to keep its surface moist.

Aqueous humor doesn't just sit there; it's continuously flowing in and out of the eye through the pupil, and is then reabsorbed into the bloodstream through a meshwork of drainage canals around the outer edge of the iris (the colored part of the eye). The usual analogy one hears about the circulation of this eye fluid is that it's like a sink with the faucet turned on. The tissues that produce the fluid are the faucets, and in order for the sink not to overflow, the draining canals of the eye (like the drain and pipes connected to the sink) must remain open and unobstructed.

The internal pressure in the eye depends on how much fluid it contains, and whether or not it can move freely in and out. As we grow older, the drainage canals tend to angle and bend, interfering with this flow. As a result, fluid backs up, stagnates, and causes increased pressure within the eye. Whether or not this ends up as glaucoma depends, to a great extent, on the height of the pressure level. This condition is called *primary open-angle glaucoma* and accounts for 90 percent of the cases of glaucoma in the elderly. It's an insidious process that rarely causes any telltale symptoms until the optic nerve has been damaged and vision is lost. The diagnosis is suggested when the doctor finds elevated pressure in the eyes, changes in the contour of the optic nerve, and, most important, alterations in your field of vision. The earliest symptoms of glaucoma are some loss of side vision; trouble adjusting when you go from a brightly lit room to a darker one; difficulty doing close work; the need to change prescriptions for glasses more frequently; and seeing colored rings around lights.

More serious but much less common is *acute-angle closure glaucoma* (to which, for some reason, Asians and Eskimos are especially prone). Instead of a gradual blockage of the drainage canals and a slow, progressive buildup of fluid pressure within the eye, the canals become obstructed suddenly. This results in a variety of acute symptoms, including blurred vision, pain in the eyes, headache, nausea and vomiting, and the appearance of rainbow haloes when you look at lights. *This is a medical emergency for which you should call your doctor immediately.* Unless it's treated quickly, blindness can occur within hours.

There are other, less common forms of glaucoma such as congenital, juvenile, and low-tension, but open-angle and acute-angle closure are the ones associated with aging.

The only way to detect increased eye pressure before it damages the optic nerve is to have regular, comprehensive eye examinations. This should include *tonometry,* in which the eye pressure is measured. (I'm sure you know that your blood pressure should be no higher than 140/80, but do you ever worry that your intraocular pressure is greater than 23 millimeters of mercury?) The drainage angle of your eye should also be evaluated (*gonioscopy*). Drops numb your eyes, and the doctor places a handheld lens on them. The lens has a mirror, which allows him or her to look sideways into your eye in order to see whether the area between the iris and the cornea is open. The status of your optic nerve is determined by *ophthalmoscopy,* and your peripheral (side) vision is tested by *perimetry.* I suggest such an exam at age thirty-five and forty; then every two to four years until you're fifty, and annually thereafter. Who should do these exams, your family doctor or an ophthalmologist? At the risk of offending some of my primary-care colleagues, I believe that the stakes are so high in this disorder that you should settle for nothing less than a specialist.

RISK FACTORS FOR GLAUCOMA

Unlike cataracts, macular degeneration, and some of the other accompaniments of aging, there's no way to prevent increased pressure within the eye. It's a roll of the biological dice whether or not you're going to develop it. But remember, although there's nothing you can do to stop your eye pressure from rising, you can prevent glaucoma blindness by lowering elevated pressure as soon as it's discovered.

Certain people are more vulnerable than others, and they should be even more compulsive about having regular, routine, and thorough eye examinations. Here are some of the risk factors:

- **Age** is the most important factor. Vulnerability starts by the time you're fifty.
- **Nearsightedness**
- **African ancestry** is important. African Americans develop glaucoma four to five times more frequently than do Caucasians, and they do so earlier too (by age thirty-five rather than after fifty years).
- **If several members of your immediate family** have glaucoma, your chances of getting it are greater than if there was no such familial predisposition.
- **Previous physical injury to the eyes** (secondary glaucoma).
- **Chronic anemia**
- **Diabetes**
- **Chronic use of steroid hormones**

If you fall into any of the above categories, you should have regular eye examinations every one to two years after age thirty-five. If you haven't had an eye exam in two years because you don't have medical insurance and can't afford it, call the Glaucoma 2001 information and Referral Line at 1-800-GLAUCOMA. They will refer you to an eye doctor in your area who will perform the first exam at no charge.

HOW TO NORMALIZE INCREASED PRESSURE WITHIN THE EYE

As I indicated earlier, glaucoma cannot be cured, but you can stop it from getting worse with the right drugs. If you are being treated for glaucoma, it's important to know what medications are available, which ones to avoid, and which are optimal for you.

There are several different kinds of eye drops and pills to treat glaucoma. Beta-blockers and carbonic anhydrase inhibitors decrease the amount of aqueous humor produced so that there is less fluid within the eye; miotics and epinephrine compounds increase the outflow of fluid from the eye. Virtually every glaucoma treatment can produce some side effects, not only in your eyes (stinging, reddening, blurring, headaches, drowsiness), but in the rest of the body as well (tingling of the fingers and toes, changes in heart rate, loss of appetite, and others). The medication your doctor prescribes for you will depend not only on the specific problem in your eyes, but on other aspects of your health as well. So make sure that your eye doctor is in touch with your primary-care physician before you begin to take any anti-glaucoma medication. For example, "beta-blocker" drugs (Timoptic, Betagan, Betimol, Betoptic, and Ocupress), though usually well tolerated, can cause confusion, depression, impotence, and other problems in persons with heart or lung disease. The "miotic" drugs, such as pilocarpine, carbachol, and phospholine iodide, make the pupils small so that less light gets into your eyes. This dims your vision, especially at night, especially if you happen also to have cataracts. These drugs may also give you a headache, which almost always clears up in a few days. The drug with the fewest side effects in the epinephrine category (it's also the most expensive) is Propine. However, epinephrine is adrenaline, and should be used very carefully, if at all, by anyone with high blood pressure, heart trouble, or pulse irregularities. "Carbonic anhydrase inhibitors" are members of the sulfa family, the prototype of which is Diamox. If you're allergic to sulfa, holler when you get this prescription. It comes in pill and drop form. The eye drops have fewer side effects than the pill, but avoid them if you're sulfa sensitive.

If your anti-glaucoma medication has been giving you unpleasant side effects, ask your doctor about two newer drugs: the "alpha-agonists" and the "prostaglandin-agonists." The former (Alphagan, Lopidine) can cause local eye symptoms such as stinging, tearing, and burning only when you first use them. In addition to lowering the intraocular pressure, they have an unexpected cosmetic bonus—they open droopy eyelids a little. The other drug (Xalatan) belongs to an entirely new class of anti-glaucoma agent that works by opening an alternate drainage pathway within the eye. All you need is one drop at bedtime. Xalatan also has an interesting cosmetic side effect—if your eyes are hazel, greenish, or blue-brown in color, it may turn them brown permanently. (So what? You can always buy a colored contact lens!)

You must take faithfully whatever medication is prescribed for glaucoma. There should be no "I forgot my medicines yesterday. I was too busy" (or stressed, or harassed, or whatever) excuses. Glaucoma is a high-stakes game in which the winner ends up with eyesight and the loser goes blind.

Laser therapy can be effective in treating some cases of open-angle glaucoma when medication has either been unsuccessful or was started too late. This procedure, in which the laser beam enlarges the angle of the ducts, is called *trabeculoplasty* and can be done in the doctor's office. In the less common acute-angle closure form of glaucoma, the laser beam creates a hole in the iris (the colored part of the eye), permitting the aqueous humor to flow more freely through it. This procedure *(iridotomy)* requires only topical or local anesthesia and can also usually be done in the ophthalmologist's office.

If medication and lasers don't relieve your glaucoma, you may be a candidate for *filtering surgery.* Using miniature instruments, the eye surgeon removes a small piece of the wall of the eye (the tough white covering called the sclera). This leaves a tiny hole through which the aqueous humor can flow, reducing the pressure in the eye. Although none of these techniques restore lost vision, they can prevent matters from getting worse.

WHAT TO REMEMBER ABOUT GLAUCOMA

1. Glaucoma is the second leading cause of blindness in the United States. It is the result of a prolonged increase in the pressure of the fluid that nourishes the

interior of the eye. There is no way to prevent this increased intraocular pressure. Left untreated, this elevated pressure can damage the optic nerve, which carries visual images to the brain.

2. The key to holding glaucoma and blindness at bay is a regular, routine, thorough eye examination by a specialist.

3. A variety of eye drops and pills can treat increased intraocular pressure. What's best for you depends on the presence or absence of other disease states or allergies.

4. When medications fail, there are several procedures that can prevent progression of vision loss. However, blindness due to glaucoma cannot be reversed.

20

FINAL REFLECTIONS

The Bottom Line

The foregoing chapters describe specific strategies for coping with the diseases or infirmities to which we become more vulnerable as we grow older. However, woven through all of them is a single thread called lifestyle—the personal mosaic that makes you the individual you are. It reflects the sum total of your habits, your outlook on life, your frame of mind, your spiritual or religious bent, and even the love you have for those around you. In my opinion, lifestyle is the main determinant of successful aging; everything else is merely a Band-Aid to existence. I'm not denying the importance of eating "right," keeping your blood pressure normal, and following the other "rules" your doctor lays down. I have enunciated them in detail in these pages. But your *attitude* toward life, and the pleasure, satisfaction, and happiness you derive from it, are critical to healthy longevity.

Aging, the path we follow from the time we're born to the day we die, is full of roadblocks called disease. The duration of our journey along that path and the quality of our lives depend on how well we deal with the obstacles that lie in wait at every bend in the road. Some, such as the progressive narrowing of critical arteries, creep up on us, while others, like the rupture of a congenital aneurysm in the brain, are sudden. Our genes may render some of these trappings of age beyond our control, but here's the good news: *You can anticipate, prevent, delay, or modify most of the others so that they don't make you sick and old before your time.*

In my many years as a doctor, I've seen hundreds of patients grow old. I've come to understand why some of them age more successfully and later in life than others do. Here are some of my observations—and my advice based on them.

1. Contentment Is a Key to Successful Aging

You cannot attain contentment by being a gourmand at the table of life, grasping for more and more and never being satiated. The *Oxford English Dictionary* defines "contentment" as the "process of being satisfied; pleasure; gratification." In my experience, your life will be "content" if you give every challenge the best shot you can, and then accept the outcome with equanimity. Ongoing bitterness, dissatisfaction, frustration, chronic anger, and envy are the handmaidens and harbingers of disease.

It's easy for me to prescribe "contentment"; filling that prescription is a different matter. It's not nearly as simple as taking a blood-pressure pill or reducing the fat in your diet. However, there are things you can do to help you achieve a sense of contentment. They include keeping physically and mentally fit by exercising regularly, and practicing several mind-body techniques.

Eastern cultures and religions have long appreciated the unity of the mind and the body. Western medical practitioners have, until quite recently, given this concept short shrift. With our newer understanding of the immune system and how it adversely responds to stress, there is a new respect for the influence of thought and emotion on physical well-being. "It's all in your head" used to be a term of disparagement. If something was "all in your head," your doctor would send you to a shrink. These days, however, enlightened doctors, of which there is a growing number, try to determine what it is that's in your head, and attempt to get rid of it. Mind-body techniques can be as effective as prolonged psychiatric care. They include t'ai chi, biofeedback, meditation, and yoga, among others. These mind-body programs are important, and I suggest you find out about them. They can help you to achieve the contentment that is necessary for healthy longevity. Following is a brief description of some of the techniques with which I am personally familiar.

Biofeedback manipulates physiological responses—breathing, blood pressure, heart rate—that normally proceed at their own pace and are not under our conscious control. Monitoring electrodes are attached to various parts of the body (depending on the physiologic process being addressed) and permit you to see how your thought processes affect them. This technique is now widely used by both complementary and conventional practitioners to reduce stress and eliminate its consequences.

Meditation was made acceptable to American doctors by the work of Herbert Benson, a Harvard physician, through his book *The Relaxation Response*. This technique requires you to detach yourself from your environment and avoid all emotions or feeling. This permits you to concentrate deeply and to experience "peace, enlightenment, and tranquillity." Although meditation is a key ingredient of yoga, it has become a useful tool in its own right. The best time to meditate is early morning, but do it whenever you have the chance. Before you start, turn off the phone. Sit quietly with your eyes closed and breathe deeply. Concentrate intensely on some object such as a candle, a flower, a word, or on your breath sounds. This replaces the thoughts and problems that have been keeping you preoccupied. Now relax your facial muscles first. Let the rest of your body become limp without slouching. Search your memory for a pleasant scene, and try to visualize it as you relax totally. As you progressively breathe more deeply for the ten to twenty minutes (once or twice a day) you meditate, you can feel your energy and equanimity restored. Do try meditating. It works. For more complete instructions on how to do it, read Dr. Benson's book.

In the minds of most people, *yoga* conjures up images of swamis, gurus, and other Eastern holy types standing on their heads. But that's not the kind of yoga practiced by my wife, my daughter, or in rehabilitation centers of American hospitals, including those run by the Veterans Administration. Yoga has three major components—posture, breathing, and meditation—and its purpose is to strengthen the body and relax the mind. The designated exercises require you to perform flowing poses that tone your muscles and increase their strength.

Members of my family and my patients who do yoga regularly love it. It leaves them physically and psychologically enhanced. If you're interested, the International Association of Yoga Therapists in Mill Valley, California can put you in touch with an instructor in your area.

I have a special interest in *t'ai chi*. Many years ago, Erich Fromm, my patient and friend, performed it regularly. He and his wife would go through the breathing exercises and the movements of this ancient martial art every morning and evening. They were among the most relaxed people I knew. I believed that Fromm's equanimity stemmed from his personal philosophy. After all, he was one of the great analysts and philosophers of our time. But he attributed his unruffled demeanor to his t'ai chi exercises. Now, many years later, my oldest son has become a t'ai chi master (the Chinese call it *sifu*). He confirms what I have read in many medical journals: that in the hospital classes he conducts, the elderly who do t'ai chi are happier people who have better balance and suffer fewer falls.

T'ai chi is a blend of the healing and martial arts whose purpose over the centuries has been physical health and spiritual strength. I understand that it sprang from the need of Chinese monks some 1,000 years ago to protect themselves against warlords and bandits. The goal of t'ai chi is to achieve harmony between the body and the mind. It helps you to derive an emotional, mental, and spiritual awareness that calms and heals. More and more hospitals and rehabilitation centers are offering t'ai chi.

2. Exercising Regularly Is Extremely Important

As soon as you're old enough to walk, you should get into the habit of exercising. The more spry and physically active you remain, the better you'll age. Don't expect to have the stamina to get up and go if you're a habitual couch potato. It doesn't take much to keep fit. Healthy exercise doesn't mean working out to the verge of collapse. Just walk, dance, swim, or do any type of aerobic exercise. Thirty minutes a day is enough to keep your heart pumping blood to your muscles and your brain. (It will also keep your weight down).

3. Avoid Being Overweight

This doesn't mean engaging in the national obsession with weight—weighing yourself religiously every day and watching every morsel you put in your mouth. Keep your weight down for medical, not cosmetic, reasons.

Let's face it: You'll probably never look like Robert Redford or Cindy Crawford. But then again, you don't have to. In the real world, thin is not necessarily beautiful. Just don't get flabby and fat.

I believe that people who limit their meat intake are generally healthier than those who don't. I also feel that the benefits of restricting animal products are more than a matter of reducing cholesterol or fat intake. I suspect that man was not made to be a carnivore. Data from many countries suggest that health and longevity are tied to the consumption of fruit, fish, grains, and vegetables. That's not to say that a delicious steak now and then will kill you. It won't, and you should have it if you enjoy it. But in my view, you're better off eating more fish, poultry, fruits, and vegetables than animal products.

4. No Smoking

What the surgeon general says about tobacco is absolutely true! I'd like to be able to tell my nicotine-addicted friends that it's really okay for them to smoke as long as they do everything else "right." Many of them would love to hear me say so because they're so full of guilt. But, as compassionate as I think I am, I cannot ignore my observations and those of doctors everywhere, that the ranks of the victims of heart attack, stroke, and cancer are filled with smokers. Tobacco accounts for hundreds of thousands of deaths each year in this country alone.

5. Limit Alcohol Intake

I have occasionally been taken to task for saying good things about alcohol—not drunkenness, but a cocktail, a bottle of beer, or a glass of wine to accompany a meal. You've read in these pages about the downside of booze, and you know how it hurts the liver, kills automobile drivers, and wrecks marriages. But you've also learned that in moderation it does good things for the heart and circulation. But don't view alcohol as a medication. If you've never had a drink, don't start now. And if you have trouble stopping when you've had enough, pack it in. But if you can limit yourself to no more than one or two drinks a day and they help you relax, have no guilt.

6. Find a Good Doctor

Ninety percent of all medical bills are run up during the last year of a person's life, so although having a good doctor is important at any age, it's especially so for older folks. What is a "good" doctor? The truth is that most primary-care physicians (remember when they used to be called "family doctors"?) have pretty much the same knowledge base. What makes one "better" than another is compassion (especially for the elderly) and availability. That's how you should choose your caregiver. The smartest doctor in the world won't do you much good if he or she is not available when needed or to whom you're just another prostate, heart, or gallbladder. And, of course, if your doctor is nihilistic about treating older persons, then find a new one. How often have I heard colleagues say, "What do you expect? He's eighty!" That attitude is all too common in hospitals, as well as among doctors and the health-care companies for whom they work. The calendar should not determine how aggressive your therapy should be. I have seen patients in their nineties undergo successful heart surgery for control of their symptoms.

Unfortunately, since there are fewer remaining solo practitioners because most doctors have been forced, by economic reasons, to join larger groups or are working for managed-care for-profit companies, your options are limited. Still, when you do have a choice, pick a doctor who knows, who cares, and who answers your calls. The best way to find one is to ask your friends and relatives. Hospitals and medical societies recommend doctors on the basis of their credentials—important, but only a small part of the story.

Once you've selected a doctor, the next thing to do, as early as your fifties, is to buy long-term health-care insurance. You're much more likely to collect on that than on your fire insurance. The need for extended care, either at home or in a nursing facility, is a reality for most people— and it's expensive. Unless you are very wealthy and can foot the bill for long-term around-the-clock care, look into buying such a policy now. The sooner you get it, the less it costs.

7. Finally, Don't Take Yourself Too Seriously

You're not indispensable. There are many more where you came from. Learn how to laugh—at yourself first. A belly laugh is the best medicine, either brand name or generic. And you can never overdose with it.

In closing, let me remind you not to sit around feeling sorry for yourself, moping about your upcoming birthday and your inexorable progression to senior status. Remember that each new birthday is proof that you're making it. It doesn't mean that you're one year closer to a fixed termination date, because the older you get, the longer you'll live. Life expectancy for a child born today is about seventy-eight years, but that estimate is based on a certain number of deaths during infancy, childhood, and adolescence. Once you've made it into adult life, your expectancy goes up. So at seventy, you can look forward not to the seventy-eight years you expected at birth, but to fifteen more years. And at ninety, you have more mileage left than you ever dreamed of when you were thirty. The older you get, the better the outlook.

Instead of ruminating about your inevitable demise, concentrate on enhancing the quality of the life you have now. Forget those images of crotchety old seniors. Don't focus on nursing homes; get your inspiration from tennis tournaments and marathons for those in their eighties. And regardless of your politics, take as your role model someone like former President Bush, who at the age of seventy-two was vigorous enough to parachute from 12,500 feet—just for the fun of it. (If he'd eaten more broccoli, he probably could have leaped from 20,000 feet!) Or Senator Glenn, who at age seventy-eight has gone into space again. And whom did President Yeltsin's doctors call when they needed another opinion about doing heart surgery on their patient? Eighty-eight-year-old Michael DeBakey, who still flies around the world, outpacing colleagues fifty years his junior.

You can have an intact mind and body even if you have some underlying illness. You can remain vigorous despite a chronic health problem, as long as you're taking care of it.

The anti-aging "formulas" for each of the disorders and symptoms discussed in the preceding chapters are relevant at every age because the aging process begins the moment you're born. Men and women in their forties and fifties should realize that "maturity" is only a hop, skip, and jump away from "old." The moment you subconsciously begin to make performance comparisons with someone in their thirties—in such areas as sports, business, and sexual performance—your anti-aging battle should begin.

No one lives forever; no doctor can tell you when you will meet your Maker. No one should die young, but by the same token, death should not be preceded by years of feeling frail, enfeebled, and infirm. So aim to make it at least well into your eighties or nineties (maybe, with a bit of luck, 100 or even slightly more), in possession of your faculties, feeling well and strong, able to enjoy each day and anticipating tomorrow's dawn with pleasure. *This objective is realistic and attainable.* Throw the calendar away. Follow these basics, live now, and you *will* grow old later.

INDEX